The Emperor is Buck Naked

Why Medical Evidence IS NOT NECESSARILY PROOF

EUGENE PAUL, MD

outskirts
press

Outskirts Press, Inc.
http://www.outskirtspress.com

Paperback ISBN: 978-1-4787-8385-5
Hardback ISBN: 978-1-4787-8514-9

Outskirts Press and the "OP" logo are trademarks belonging to Outskirts Press, Inc.

PRINTED IN THE UNITED STATES OF AMERICA

Table of Contents

Acknowledgements

This book was written in virtual isolation, and that may explain some of the obvious flaws. Prior to beginning this, my first book, I read much about how one should go about writing a work of nonfiction. I read that one should not avoid sending at least portions of the developing manuscript to impartial reviewers. Nonetheless, I ignored the advice - perhaps as much out of arrogance as insecurity. Whatever criticisms are offered, I will probably take under consideration. I will, no doubt, write a better book the next time. Having sought the advice of few in terms of how I should write this book, I have very few to thank....and as a consequence of that fact, no one to blame but myself. There are, nonetheless, a few to whom I am most indebted, and I have listed them in this section.

There is my editor, Susan Settlage, whom I knew little about except what could be gleaned from a resume and one telephone conversation. Essentially, I took a chance and lucked out big time. Brilliantly, she made subtle changes to the text - so subtle, in fact, that it seemed that little had been altered. yet, the syntax and readability was obviously much improved. She helped me check and (in some cases) find more appropriate reference materials. Again, Susan, I thank you.

I am grateful to my fellow music lover, longtime student of the trumpet and friend, Larry Divack of Little Neck. He provided constant encouragement and thoughtful conversation while I prepared the manuscript for more than three years while working full time. He also offered meaningful suggestions for a few of the early chapters, and I am most appreciative of those contributions.

During April 2010, when I was pissing and moaning about having left New York City for Atlanta , my youngest daughter, Dalila, provided me with the encouraging, grown-up advice that enabled me to get started on the writing and dispense with the whining. I thank you, D.

My older daughter, Dara, presented me with essential advice that helped me get basic things done simply and quickly on the computer. Without her, I would have likely - due to impatience - hired a team of computer geeks.

My son and first born, Eugene, conveyed constant interest and encouragement while I wrote this book. He also offered positive reinforcement by critiquing some of the early chapters.

Finally (and most significantly) I thank my friend and companion for more than fifty years. She has always supported me in the most important ventures in my life - whether they seemed like pipe dreams or realistic goals. She is the one who has always had my back, with or without a smile: my wife of now fifty years, Birdie. Thank you for ALL that you do.

Introduction

I wrote this essay after almost 40 years of trying to understand and become a better practitioner of clinical medicine. This discipline involves listening to the patient's account of what ails them, an exercise that is referred to as taking a history. This is usually followed by performing a physical examination and obtaining various tests to get some ideas as to the cause of their complaints. The goal is to provide a cure — when possible or, at least, — relief of symptoms. The hope is to provide some understanding that may help avoid or minimize the likelihood of disease complications or recurrence.

This book is certainly not for everyone; it is not meant primarily for the medically or scientifically trained. I accept that it may be of little interest to the vast majority of individuals who are content with sheepishly following the authoritative ORDERS of their health care providers without question. It is aimed at the proactive man or woman of any age; the intelligent non-professional who is interested in taking primary responsibility for their own health, perhaps with the *assistance* of their medical professionals, who should be thought of as their consultants. Here, I am speaking of individuals not involved in an immediately life threatening situation, in which case, it is understood that the medical professional would appropriately assume the primary role in medical or surgical management. Hopefully, this book also will be of use to the medical professional in training; be they student physicians or so-called mid level providers, *e.g.* Physician Assistants (PAs) and Nurse Practitioners. For whoever has the responsibility of directly caring for patients should be aware of the thin ice upon which they are often skating in terms of what we absolutely know.

Whether you are professional listening to some professor of medicine at a conference speaking self assuredly about the latest recommendations for the treatment of heart disease, diabetes, cancer, or part of a general audience listening to a radio or television guru pontificating about what foods to eat, herbs or supplements to take to prevent any and all afflictions or even if you find ourselves surfing the internet for "natural" substances to help you remain forever young, we may find their statements glibly made and always *presumably* backed by "solid scientific evidence." One of the most often used phrases we hear from these experts and other stuffed shirts is, "the data clearly shows that ......blah, blah, blah." Meanwhile the intended audience rarely has a clue as to what the data or studies actually mean. The data could be absolute and unmitigated BS and most would be none the wiser.

This book was written to give the intelligent general reader or student some perspective. One of the inherent fallacies, as implied by the adulation which is often given to "data" or evidence, is the presumption that *medicine* is, in fact, *hard science*, as we generally understand it. We assume that the studies represent a consistently reliable representation of the real world of human beings; those who do not participate in these studies. The investigation of human beings does not lend itself neatly to the experimentation common to the biology or chemistry laboratory. The indirect evidence for the existence of subatomic particles offered by the use of the accelerator is of no use in the world of the clinician. The complexity of the anatomy and physiology (structure and function) of humans is awe-inspiring in itself. Now consider the real and potential influences of genetics; the historical, and socio-political factors that can play a role in an individual's life; and the cultural milieu in which one lives, and here the extraordinary complexity of men and women becomes unfathomable. Given all of these intangibles in the study of human beings, it should be apparent that the essence of wisdom involves a greater appreciation of uncertainty and the recognition of a greater need for humility.

This book is divided into 11 relatively brief chapters. Because everyone from government officials to TV personalities continually invoke the mantra of scientific medicine, I thought it would be appropriate to begin with a discussion as to what is science, and the scientific method. Chapter two offers a brief history of what has become known as evidence-based medicine and a discussion of what, if anything, it has to do with science. Chapter three is concerned with the testing that is used in research to establish whether the results obtained are due to the objects of the investigation or due to chance. Chapter four suggests the need of some medical professionals to make bold (seemingly faith-based) assumptions in order to generalize from the specific findings in a study to the larger population. The following four chapters are concerned with a few areas of controversy, some more than others — prostate, and breast cancer screening; recommendations for some of the more popular universal vaccinations; and finally, a discussion of the lipid hypothesis. This last area is almost universally accepted in this country; that cholesterol is the prime culprit in the development of atherosclerosis and a principle cause of heart attack and stroke. Chapter nine addresses alternative medicine. Chapter 10 discusses our apparent need for certainty in medicine and I conclude in chapter 11 with a recognition that while certainty is probably universally sought after, in the real world, it is rarely achievable. Therefore, in the interest of common sense (why call it common?) and truly patient centered health care, it would behoove those of us in the medical profession to become less dogmatic and to learn and practice the virtue of humility.

My modest hope is that this book will contribute to the growing number of skeptics who take nothing for granted, question everything and take delight in the deflation of wind bags, however exalted or revered. The ultimate goal is not to become contrarian for its own sake, but rather to learn to take greater personal responsibility for our own minds and bodies in order to enjoy a fuller, self-actualized life and not one forever crippled by managed fear. This fear is enhanced by the constant publication of contradictory, non-generalizable studies and a robust pharmaceutical industry which — through its direct marketing to the general public — would have us believe that we are all suffering from one or another product deficiency.

"It aint't necessarily so." - George Gershwin

CHAPTER 1

The Scientific Method: What is it?

IT IS IMPORTANT to recognize that there is no one way to conduct science. There is often variability and overlap in the steps by which investigators proceed. Therefore the description that follows may appear text bookish and bare only a superficial resemblance to how real scientists conduct their day to day business. Having offered this qualification we can then say that by science, we typically imply the systematic study of the natural world, of which there are several subdivisions; among them biology, chemistry, astronomy, geology and physics, for example. Its roots can be found in Babylonia and Egypt and its development in Greece and Rome. Science is traditionally defined by its unique method of "truth-finding," by its "scientific method." The method involves careful observation, resulting in the development of preliminary explanations based on limited evidence, which is called an hypothesis. This is followed by experimentation to test the hypothesis and further observation with the generation of additional hypotheses.

Before we answer the question as to exactly what is science; what is the scientific method, a few words are in order to explain what science is not. It is not philosophy, or religion, or metaphysics. It cannot answer questions as to why we are here, what is the purpose of life, or whether there is a creator, benevolent or otherwise. These are questions beyond the realm of science. Science says nothing about how we should behave, or what constitutes correct and moral behavior. The philosopher, Karl Popper states that a proposition is scientific if and only if, it is falsifiable (1). In other words, questions regarding the existence and nature of God, or the meaning of life cannot be proven wrong; therefore, they are not "falsifiable." This does not argue for the existence of God. It only claims that it is not a question for science. Scientific questions, on the other hand, may never be verified; or definitely proven correct, but they can be tested and refuted or falsified. Popper contends that throughout history, science has progressed by successfully proposing theories that were able to falsify previously existing theories (2). The new theory may replace the old because it does a better job of explaining some previously unknown or misunderstood phenomenon.

Using the above definition of science, the discipline predates recorded history. In keeping with the Eurocentism of western academia, it is presumed that the first scientists were a handful of Greeks, most notably Anaxagoras, who was born in Ionia, the western coast of present day Turkey. He was reportedly born approximately 500 years before the Christian era. In his work, *Anaxagoras and the Birth of the Scientific Method*, Daniel E. Gershenson credits Anaxagoras with saying that the sole purpose of life is to observe and ponder natural phenomena and to attempt to explain it rationally (3). Anaxagoras is credited with being one of the first, if not, the first, to attempt to explain the workings of nature in rational, non-religious terms. Before the Greek began his investigations, thinkers tended to attribute natural phenomena to the work of gods, spirits and other supernatural beings.

As noted above, science actually predates history and history, for all intents, begins with recorded history, *i.e.* writing. The first known writing systems were those of the Egyptians and Babylonians in the Nile Valley and Tigris-Euphrates regions, respectively. In his very useful little book, *Greek and Roman Science*, Don Nardo acknowledges that because the early Greeks were very much influenced by these earlier people, the story of Greek and Roman science must begin in Egypt and Babylonia (4). Even Herodotus, who presumptuously has been designated by western academia as "the father of history" recognized the primary role of the Egyptians, particularly in the realm of astronomy. Again quoting Nardo, "in his histories, Herodotus states that the Egyptians discovered the solar system and were the first to divide it into 12 parts — and in my opinion their method of calculation is better than the Greeks" (5).

Herodotus reportedly visited Egypt in the 5th century B.C., after which he recorded his observations concerning Egyptian science. He was not the only thinker of antiquity to recognize the African contribution. Don Nardo observes further that there are also anecdotal accounts that Thales and Pythagoras also visited Egypt. These anecdotes illustrate that these early Greek scholars were aware of and influenced by their scientific predecessors in the "Near East."(6).

Senegalese anthropologist and physicist, Cheik Anta Diop observed in 1985 in the *Nile Valley Civilizations* that Pythagoras and his disciples had been so much influenced by Egypt that, in spite of the fact that they spoke a different language and had a different writing system, they used Egyptian hieroglyphic signs in their pre-algebraic mathematical notation (7). Diop notes further that most of the scientists who provided Greece with its scientific legacy were persecuted, driven out of their native land where they fled to Egypt. Many of them went to Egypt for training, including the previously mentioned Anaxagoras, as well as Socrates, Plato and Aristotle.

Perhaps the greatest contribution of Egypt to science, ironically given our thesis, was in the field of applied science, *i.e.* medicine. Historians and archeologists have documented these contributions through an examination of the various medical papyri. The English word paper is derived from papyrus, a thick, paper-like material produced from the papyrus plant that grew in the Nile delta. The Egyptians apparently felt the need to develop a medium upon which to write that replaced stone. Papyrus was used from approximately 4000 years before the Christian era to the 11th century A.D. (8). Seven papyri concerning medicine are known to have survived. Each consists of several pages of diagnoses and treatments for medical and surgical (mostly due to trauma) problems of the day, in addition to the Kahuhn papyrus that offered gynecological treatments.

According to the Academic press *Dictionary of Science and Technology*, science is defined as the systematic observation of natural events and conditions in order to discover "*facts*"(italics mine) and to formulate laws and principles based on these facts (9). The main goal or purpose of science is to gather or collect the facts alluded to above. This is often referred to as "data." Further, the purpose of obtaining this data is to develop a deeper understanding of the natural world, the only world that we know. Ideally, science, unlike religion or politics, does not or should not deal in dogma; however, recognizing that scientists certainly can be dogmatic, they too can be wedded to paradigms. The purpose of reviewing these idealized and admittedly mechanistic definitions of science is precisely because the discipline is traditionally defined by its method. In so far as the contemporary thought leaders in medicine; popular and academic maintain that their recommendations are based upon science, it would follow that if they are doing science, they are using a recognized scientific method.

With respect to method, as Popper discussed, with his falsification criteria for what distinguished scientific from non-scientific activity, he was describing what *ought* to be. Thomas Kuhn, on the other hand, in *The Structure of Scientific Revolutions* (10) (which is an actual history of science), described his view of how science was *actually* done. Kuhn maintained that scientists operated within a particular framework, a paradigm, which is a theoretical model, a way of viewing the world. This framework influenced the way they viewed and interpreted data. More often than not , they will resist attempts at falsification. Changing paradigms is not easy because it involves taking an unorthodox position, alienating colleagues and jeopardizing reputations and funding sources. This is usually the case, what Kuhn describes as "normal" science. On occasion there are mavericks; the Galileos, Newtons, and Einsteins, whose research reveals unexpected results. Kuhn calls these results, which persistently resist conventional explanation, anomalies. When anomalies persist, we have a crisis in science that can then lead to revolution or an overhaul of an existing paradigm and its replacement. Several books have been written by and about the ideas of Popper and Kuhn. These few words, therefore, represents a gross oversimplification. My purpose here is just to illustrate that even within the so-called hard sciences, there is significant disagreement as to how the discipline is actually conducted. This will be of even greater importance as we examine how an even less precise activity such as clinical research, which deals with real human beings rather than abstract numbers, is used to make sweeping statements and recommendations regarding human beings.

In the ideal, the practice of science is not fearful of being proven wrong; it seeks only to increase our understanding of natural phenomena. It is not interested in promoting gurus or saviors; it only wants to know what *is*, what is so. Once again, this is certainly true of science, but the behavior of scientists, with their egos, insecurities, warts and all, are generally less noble. For the purposes of our examination, I am particularly fond of a definition of science offered by Nobel Prize winning physicist, Richard Feynman, who stated in, *The Pleasure of Finding Things Out* (11), "that science alone of all the subjects contains within itself the lesson of the danger of belief in the infallibility of the greatest teachers in the preceding generation." Doing science is also involves a recognition and appreciation of the fallibility of experts.

Readers, keep this definition upper most in your mind as we discuss the pretensions of many "thought leaders " in medicine later in the book.

The title of this first chapter poses a simple enough question, but the answer can take anywhere from a few lines to an entire book. There will undoubtedly be several people who would find fault with the definition. Science is often, perhaps artificially, divided into the so-called "hard" and "soft" categories. Hard science tends to refer to, for example, biology, chemistry, physics, earth science and their numerous subdivisions. Soft science more often refers to the social sciences, including psychology, sociology, political science, and economics. In his *A Beginners Guide To Scientific Method*, Stephen Carey states that, "it is sometimes said that only the hard sciences are "exact" and this is generally taken to mean that predictions about human behavior cannot hope to be as precise as, say predictions about what will happen to a gas under a specific set of conditions"(12). Therefore grand unifying principles as sought after by scientists from Anaxagoras to Einstein appear most unlikely in the soft sciences. It is said that Einstein was working on such a principle shortly before his death. The whole soft and hard dichotomy appears needlessly elitist. Suffice it to say that human behavior is far too complex and impacted by so many forces to be reduced to simple unifying principles

Lest we be misled into believing that hard science is necessarily mechanistic, precise and objective, Henry Bauer observes in his *Scientific Literacy and the Myth of The Scientific Method*, "science is both a social activity and an intellectual one. The prevailing scientific worldview is not a single, logically coherent entity so much as a mosaic of the beliefs of many specialized little scientific groups; and a belief gets incorporated in the mosaic if there is a scientific group espousing that belief"(13).

The hallmark of the scientific approach, again in the ideal, involves a healthy respect for skepticism. At its best, it does not work *for* the government, private corporations or the pharmaceutical industry, although its practitioners may be employed in those settings. Its function, its purpose is further understanding, to investigate reality as we know it and let the chips fall where they may. The danger of science, in the hands of some, however, is that it can become scripture, the new religion, as it were. As a child, when I asked the nun who taught Sunday school at St. Paul's Catholic Church in East Harlem, "Sister, but where did God come from?" she replied glibly, "God always was and always will be." Presumably she found this more comforting than simply admitting, "I don't know." Clearly, ingrained dogma serves very useful purposes, psychologically if nothing else. Hopefully we will not be content with dismissing a similar question by replying that matter and energy always were and always will be. The continuous evolution in scientific thinking and discovery mandates that we maintain a sense of humility in what we think we know at this juncture, a theme I will reiterate, hopefully not *ad nauseum*, throughout this discussion, especially as it relates to the recommendations which we make to our patients.

Now a word concerning language. It would appear that each discipline, be it medicine, law, science, or philosophy, has its own language, its own way of expressing itself. The purpose of this language is not always to communicate clearly to a broad audience, or to inform, but frequently to obfuscate, to prevent the general public from accessing precisely what they are speaking about. The fear seems to be that if anyone can understand what they are talking about, then somehow the discipline looses its specialness. Hence the need for the "specialist" to decode the invariable "word salad" that passes for discourse. Admittedly, this may be more characteristic of the legal profession than some of the other disciplines mentioned above. Therefore, part of my challenge over the next several pages will be to explain some very important concepts simply without being simple-minded, at least not excessively.

References Cited

1. Popper, K.R., *The Logic of Scientific Discovery*. New York: Routledge, 2002. p.62.
2. Ibid. p.278-279.
3. Gershenson, D.E. and D.A. Greenberg, *Anaxagoras and the Birth of Scientific Method*. 1st ed. A Blaisdell book in the history of science. New York: Blaisdell Pub. Co., 1964. p.3.
4. Nardo, D., *Greek and Roman Science*. World history series. San Diego, CA: Lucent Books, 1998. p.13.
5. Ibid.
6. Ibid. p.14.
7. Diop, C., *Africa's Contribution to World Civilization: The Exact Sciences*. Nile Valley Civilizations, 1985, p. 69.
8. Nunn, J.F., *Ancient Egyptian Medicine*. Norman: University of Oklahoma Press, 1996. p. 24-41.
9. Morris, C.G., *Academic Press Dictionary of Science and Technology*. San Diego: Academic Press. 1992.
10. Kuhn, T.S., *The Structure of Scientific Revolutions*. 3rd ed. Chicago, IL: University of Chicago Press, 1996.
11. Feynman, R.P. and J. Robbins, *The Pleasure of Finding Things Out: The Best Short Works of Richard P. Feynman*. Cambridge, Mass.: Perseus Books, 1999.
12. Carey, S.S., *A Beginner's Guide to Scientific Method*. 3rd ed. Belmont, CA: Thomson/Wadsworth, 2004.
13. Bauer, H.H., *Scientific Literacy and the Myth of the Scientific Method*. Urbana, Ill: University of Illinois Press, 1992.

CHAPTER 2

Evidence-Based Medicine: A Brief History

A WORKING DEFINITION of Evidence-Based Medicine (EBM) and one used by David Sackett, one of the premier personalities in its history and development is this: EBM is the conscientious, explicit and judicious use of the current best evidence combined with clinical expertise and patient values to make decisions about the care of individual patients (1). This definition represents EBM, at its best, worthy of respect and a concept with which few would find fault. It is all-inclusive, and respects the value of science and the judgment of clinicians, which often comes from several years of experience with perhaps thousands of patients. It also takes into account the primary player, the one for whom we are supposed to be working, the patient. However, although the patient's values may be openly respected, if they simply will not do what we advise, the message, though well camouflaged, is often "I'm the doctor here, I went to medical school, and I know what I'm doing, where did you go to medical school, and I advise the following..." Obviously, the tone would rarely be so crass and insulting, but the implication is the same. The reality is a more authoritarian and less egalitarian approach than is advertised by the standard definition of EBM. EBM is often said to represent a "structured approach to literature evaluation, leading to decisions that are based upon probability"(2). In truth, the clinician who has the responsibility of caring for the patient may rarely take this approach to the literature. This could be due to a lack of time to read the literature carefully (less than 1 hour per week by physicians in Britain and the US (3) or because many non-academic physicians lack the ability to successfully navigate through the statistics in most studies to adequately determine the strength of the reported findings. Therefore, clinicians may rely on drug salespersons (known as "reps") or presentations from experts at conferences, which are themselves greatly financed by drug companies. Several of us have time only to read the summaries or conclusions published in the various medical trade journals; most of these pages are filled with advertisements from drug and medical equipment manufacturing companies. Hence, effective influence peddling is more real than imagined.

In her examination of EBM, Jeanne Daly tells us that "In 1979, British physician Archie Cochrane reviewed the use of the randomized clinical trial and proposed that each medical specialty should identify all the trials done in its field and then prepare up-to-date, critical summaries of the relevant ones, so that practitioners would have easy access to information on effective care"(4). In the above, the operative word is *relevant*. There is very little to prevent the development of an elitist closed shop that simply does not consider studies outside of the orthodox EBM community. This is not an attempt to nitpick, but rather to again illustrate the unavoidable fallibility of the endeavor and the consequent need to avoid dogmatism when making recommendations as to what constitutes effective care.

We tend to assume, almost intuitively, that there is strength, in fact even truth, in numbers. We often insist that our recommendations for intervention or lack thereof, be evidence-based; however, it should be appreciated that there are often evidenced-based arguments for either side of a decision, depending, of course, on what one chooses to accept as evidence. The evidence which we generally want to see is large, randomized clinical trials or better, systematic reviews of several large trials; however, clinical medicine is concerned primarily with the needs of individuals, who may have little more in common with the participants of those trials than demographics (gender or race, for example). Robert Fletcher, former co-editor of the *Annals of Internal Medicine* summed up the dilemma as follows: "Good clinicians think of their patients as individuals, each a unique combination of genetic endowment, social and physical environment, past experiences, and current preferences. In contrast, randomized controlled trials are about average results in groups of patients. It's a bad match. There is no perfect solution to this dilemma," (as quoted by Jeanne Daly in *Evidence-based Medicine and the Search for a Clinical Science* (5).

The term Evidence-Based Medicine, although commonly used since the 1970s and popularized since the 1990s with David Sackett's group at McMaster University in Canada, actually had its origins, as a concept in the 11th century with the work of Persian polymath, Abdullah Ibn Sina, better known in the West as Avicenna. He lived from approximately 980 to 1037 CE. He reportedly wrote 450 treatises of various lengths on a wide range of subjects, of which 240 have survived. Some 40 of these works concentrate on medicine; the most famous of which is *The Book of Healing* and *The Canon of Medicine*. He is often regarded as the "father" of early modern medicine primarily because of his discovery of the contagious nature of infectious diseases (6). He introduced the concept of the quarantine to limit the spread of disease. In addition, he was said to initiate the use of the efficacy test, especially as it relates to clinical pharmacology (drug therapy). In *The Canon of Medicine*, he stipulates the rules for assessing the efficacy of new drugs, some of which still form the basis of modern clinical pharmacology. For example,

1. The drug must be used on a specific, simple, not composite disease.
2. The time of action of the drug must be observed so that the primary and accidental effects are not confused.
3. The effect of the drug must be seen to occur repeatedly or in several cases, for if this does not happen, it can be determined to be an accidental effect.
4. The experimentation must be done with the human body, for testing a drug on a lion or horse (animal testing) might not prove anything about the effect on humans (7).

After Avicenna, discussions in the literature of experimental medicine centered on the need to provide evidence for efficacy to improve patient care. An example is found in 18th century Europe, beginning with James Lind (1716–1794) and the treatment of scurvy. Scurvy is a disease that we now realize is caused by a deficiency of Vitamin C, also known as ascorbic acid. This substance enables our bodies to produce collagen, which builds the connective tissue that holds bones, muscles and organs together. Without Vitamin C, we would literally fall apart. The disease is characterized by swelling and bleeding of the gums, fever, exhaustion, bleeding into the skin, feelings of paralysis and ultimately death. Vitamin C is found in a variety of fruits and vegetables and, therefore, few of us need be concerned about scurvy these days. However, during the 16th to 18th century, it was a major cause of death, particularly among sailors because of their prolonged periods of service aboard ship with their restricted diets. In 1747, Lind, a Scottish physician serving on a British battleship, suspected that there might be a dietary cause for the disease. He was familiar with the 16th century account of several Portuguese sailors suffering from the disabling effects of scurvy who, when their ship passed through a Caribbean island, requested that they be put ashore so that they could at least die on land. Reportedly, when the same ship revisited the island a year later, the men aboard were shocked to see their old comrades alive and seemingly healthy. They had apparently survived by eating the fruits and vegetables that grew on the island, which they named Curacao, the Portuguese word for cure. Being aware of this history, Lind decided to conduct what is considered to be the world's first recorded clinical trial. He chose 12 of the sickest sailors aboard his ship and divided them into six groups of two persons each. He offered a different treatment for each group; *i.e.* vinegar, garlic paste, seawater, sulfuric acid and lemons or oranges. He noted that the group treated with the fruits recovered whereas the others did not. Despite the very dramatic results in this small trial, it still took another 50 years before the British Navy mandated the provision of lime juice for each of its sailors (8).

While not a medical investigator, British physician, Thomas Beddoes (1760–1808) provided the theoretical basis or rationale for what was to become Evidence-Based Medicine in the 20th century. Beddoes believed that the medicine of his day was secretive, ill informed and dangerous (9). In a published letter of 1808, he outlined his recommendations for reform. He advised that physicians working in hospitals and clinics collect all medical facts related to the care of patients and the outcomes of treatment and that these facts be transferred to a central location or board within the United Kingdom. He recommended that seminars be held regularly whereby all practitioners could share this information. He further advised that physicians publish their experiences and findings regularly. Beddoes believed that the very life of the population depended on the sharing of this information. The ideas of Thomas Beddoes predated by over 150 years the development of an international network for identifying and systematizing medical evidence, primarily through randomized-clinical trials, made available to all practitioners, patients and their advocates. This was the brain-child of physician and epidemiologist, Archie Cochrane and is now known as The Cochrane Library (10).

The next significant figure to appear in the history of EBM was

19th century French physician, Pierre Louis (1787-1872). As a result of his work on the wards of Charité Hospital in Paris, he published his studies in a series of monographs, the most notable of which was the 1836 work, *Researches in Phthisis* (which was the old name for tuberculosis). The findings were based on autopsy dissections of 358 patients and was said to be the first time that anyone had counted cases and classified the outcome of the treatments. His statistical analysis was said to be the first of its kind. Louis also provided a statistical analysis of typhoid fever, distinguished it from typhus and gave the former its name. Incidentally, typhoid is caused by a bacterium of the salmonellae family and is spread when the organism gets into the food or water via an infected person. Typhus is caused when an insect such as a flea or louse is infected with bacteria in the rickettsii family and bites a human being. Louis also is credited with publishing a severe condemnation of bloodletting, documenting its lack of efficacy for virtually every condition for which it was prescribed (10). This was a medical approach that was practiced throughout the world for approximately 2,000 years. The rationale behind the practice was based on the ancient notion that blood and other body fluids were substances, "humors," which required proper balancing to maintain good health. This "treatment" was recommended for a myriad of conditions including acne, asthma, cancer, diabetes, epilepsy and many more. It is said that George Washington requested bloodletting for his throat infection in 1799, had close to 2 quarts removed and died soon thereafter (11). It would behoove those among us who think these practices absurd to temper our ridicule as we have the benefit of 200 years of hindsight. It appears to be a truism that today's science is often tomorrow's quackery. One can only wonder what will be said of many of our current "evidence-based therapies" 50 to 100 years from now.

Today we take it for granted that health care providers should wash their hands if going from one patient to another, however, this was not always the case. In 1846 an Austrian Physician, Ignaz Simmelweis

(1818–1865) was working at Vienna General Hospital, reportedly one of the major obstetrical institutions in Europe. While there, he made some extraordinary observations about maternal and infant illness and death. He noted that there were a great many more deaths among women who delivered in the hospital than those who delivered at home. Also, the babies in the hospital died of the same diseases as their mothers. In addition, he noted that a greater number of deaths occurred at one clinic compared to a second clinic. Therefore, he set out to find an explanation for the differences in mortality. He was able to eliminate from consideration factors that we would now refer to as confounders, *i.e.* the birthing positions of the women, their different locations in the hospital and their social or economic class. He noticed that the women from the clinic that had the higher mortality used physicians and medical students, whereas the others used midwives. It was common practice for the physicians and students to go directly from the autopsy to the delivery rooms and perform vaginal examinations on the women in labor. The midwives, however, did not perform autopsies. He, therefore, correctly conjectured that the physicians were transmitting infectious organisms from the cadavers to the women. He then instituted a policy of hand washing with lime by anyone performing autopsies who would then examine women in labor. After beginning the policy, the mortality rate of the first clinic soon decreased to that of the second (8). This was not an intricate or sophisticated trial, but it demonstrated what could be accomplished by an astute physician who conducted an experiment with a control group at one clinic and a treatment group at the other, the results of which was of huge clinical significance, a concept which we will discuss further in subsequent chapters.

The Medical Research Council (MRC) of the United Kingdom was set up in 1911 primarily to address the global epidemic of tuberculosis (TB), which was, at the time the leading cause of death of young adults in Europe and North America. TB, an infectious disease most commonly involving the lungs and spread from one person to another by the respiratory route (coughing or sneezing), had no reliably effective medical treatment prior to the 1940s. The antibiotic, streptomycin, was developed in the United States in 1944. Laboratory testing proved the drug to be effective against the organism responsible for the disease, the tubercle bacillus. For this reason, a trial was conducted to test the efficacy of treatment in human beings in 1948 (12). There were 107 people in the trial. One group representing the control was treated only with bed rest, which was the standard of care at the time; the treatment group was given streptomycin in addition to bed rest. Neither the patients nor the physicians reviewing the monthly chest x-rays were aware of which group the patients were assigned to. The study was therefore said to be blinded. The trial was concluded after 15 months. The treatment was assessed as being effective. There were 12 deaths among the treatment group and 24 among the controls, however, drug resistance, a common problem with the use of antibiotics, where the drug becomes less effective in killing the organism, was noted in the vast majority of treated patients. Also, the rate of clinical deterioration was noted to be greater in the control group. Despite the small sample size, and the relatively modest results, this trial was nonetheless, considered a landmark in that it ushered in the modern era of randomized clinical trials and served as a model for subsequent experiments to prove the efficacy of drug treatment.

In 1972, the U.S. Congress created the Office of Technology Assessment (OTA) to provide the members of Congress and its committees with ideally objective expert analysis of new scientific issues of the day including technologies utilized in healthcare. During the 23 years of its existence it produced several hundred studies on a wide range of issues including health care, acid rain and climate change. The agency was abolished in 1995 by the Republican controlled 104th Congress as part of its "Contract with America," which advocated reducing the size and expense of government. The OTA was deemed unnecessary as it was said to be duplicative, performing a function that could and was being provided by other agencies (13). In 1986, the Institute of Medicine's Council on Health Care Technology was established "to promote the development and application of technology assessment in health care and to review health care technologies for their appropriate use" (14). However, the organization lost public funding in 1989. In the 1990s the Agency For Health Care Policy and Research was developed to focus on clinical guidelines. It was in this decade that EBM was really developed as a way to improve and evaluate patient care.

Just as the hospital was long regarded as "the doctor's workshop," the physician's word was perceived as golden. But increasingly the physician's expertise no longer went unquestioned. It was no longer sufficient for an experienced clinician to assert "in my clinical judgment," in providing a rationale for clinical decisions. It was increasingly recognized that one physician's clinical experience or judgment may or may not be relevant in another clinical setting. David Sackett, a Chicago native, trained in internal medicine and kidney disease, later realized the need to develop greater skills in epidemiology and public health and soon after studied at the Harvard School of Public health. After spending time in the department of medicine at the University of Buffalo, he was eventually invited to McMaster University in Canada and the rest, as they say, is history (at least in the world of EBM). It was in an editorial in 1996 in the British Medical Journal that Sackett offered the definition of EBM with which we opened this chapter.

The proponents of EBM cannot be held responsible for the approach failing to do what it was not designed to do. We cannot blame its advocates for its abuses who, for example, may be more concerned with reducing health care costs, irrespective of its impact on health care delivery. There are, however, several legitimate criticisms that have been offered. First, it has now been 23 years since Gordon Guyatt coined the term EBM, 17 years since Sackett offered a formal definition and, ironically, by its own criteria, there is little or no evidence that EBM actually improves patient care. Several papers begin with the generally accepted definition of EBM offered by Sackett or the expanded interpretation by former *Annals of Internal Medicine Editor*, Frank Davidoff (15) and then go on to intuitively express the belief that patients are better served by physicians who practice EBM than those who don't, but *proof* is never forthcoming. Secondly, it is often stated that the definition of "evidence" is too narrowly defined. The gold standard of proof is presumed to be the randomized clinical trial. This drastically limits the type of questions that can be answered because of the costs (millions in the larger trials) and length of time it takes to conduct the trials. In statistics "power equations" are used to determine at the outset how many patients must be enrolled in the study in order to see a significant difference in the groups studied. Therefore, if the study population is not large enough, it may be said to lack sufficient power to draw inferences from the results. It could be argued that physicians have always used "evidence" to determine treatment approaches. Their evidence, however, may have been based upon their understanding of the pathophysiological process of the patient's disease or complaint in question. They may have been using the "evidence" provided by 20 to 30 years of experience with patients with similar complaints. As we alluded to above, who's to say their evidence is less reliable in providing care for their particular patient than that obtained from the results of a randomized trial. We have only, it seems, the "faith" of the EBM practitioner that findings in the randomized group of strangers somehow have relevance to this individual that you have before you. This is an old, and some would say, tired complaint, but no less valid. More will be said about the dangers of extrapolating, or taking this leap of faith, in chapter 4. The limitations of science are often not appreciated. We are often impressed with science because of its alleged rigor, which is strengthened by numbers. Numbers provides greater legitimacy. Numbers are *hard*, feelings are *soft*. Therefore, the numbers of statistics impress and mesmerize us, especially as few of us understand the peculiar speech of the statistician. Doctors are no exception. Few doctors have had any formal training in statistics, beyond possibly, an introductory course. So frequently, what we don't understand, we tend to revere. This may be particularly true for the less experienced physician. EBM uses the language of statistics, which makes inferences about populations and, again, we are not dealing with populations in the office. In his definition of EBM, Davidoff boldly and perhaps arrogantly proclaims, "identifying the best evidence means using epidemiological and biostatistical ways of thinking" (16). Good luck with proving that.

The randomized trial, while possibly the single best instrument to allow for reliable generalization, is, when taken in isolation, inherently and seriously flawed. The process of randomization may be incapable of detecting fundamental differences between the study and control population; such as genetic differences, and anatomical differences that could only be detected by subjecting the participants to invasive, expensive and risky procedures such as catherizations, biopsies, *etc*. Therefore, when the results are analyzed and small but statistically significant differences are found, the investigators will tend to assign greater importance to these small differences than is warranted. So many medical and quasi-medical types when making recommendations to patients in the office or to the general public on TV or radio are quick to site "all the studies" which support their bias, however, an uninformed public has no way of appreciating just how flawed and unreliable these recommendations are as they are often based upon instruments (trials) that are themselves tainted. This is not to say that the trials should not be done or results from them be summarily ignored. The point is that the trial should not be regarded as sacrosanct. We should regard it as just one more piece of evidence to include in our review as we proceed to make recommendations. Here, I will introduce a common theme that bares repeating multiple times; that is the need for greater humility in a world filled with uncertainty. All knowledge is, at best, contingent and the purpose of science is to increase our understanding of just how things are, how they really work, but without dogma. This point is not a concern reserved for the philosopher. On the contrary, dogma has to be resisted by all of us, because virtually everything we do, every piece of advice we follow coming from doctors or media pundits and personalities is based upon presumptions of a certainty that does not and usually cannot exist.

References Cited

1. Sacket, D.L., Rosenburg, W.M., Gray, J.A., Haynes, R.B. and Richardson, W.S., Evidence based medicine: what it is and what it isn't. *British Medical Journal*, 1996. **312**(2023): p. 71-72.
2. Turlik, M., Introduction to evidence based medicine. *The Foot and Ankle Journal*, 2009. **2**(2).
3. Saint, S., D.A. Christakis, S. Saha, J.G. Elmore, D.E. Welsh, P. Baker, and T.D. Koepsell, Journal Reading Habits of Internists. *Journal of General Internal Medicine*, 2000. **15**(12): p. 881-884.
4. Daly, J., *Evidence-based Medicine and the Search for a Science of Clinical Care*. Vol. 12: Univ of California Press. 2005. p.154.
5. Ibid. p.227.
6. Goodman, L.E., *Avicenna*. Cornell University Press. 2006.
7. Avicenna, L. Bakhtiar, O.C. Gruner, M.H. Shah, and J.R. Crook, *The Canon of Medicine*. Chicago, Ill: KAZI Publ, 1999.
8. Greenstone, G., The roots of evidence-based medicine. *British Columbia Medical Journal*, 2009. **51**(8): p. 342-344.
9. Goodman, N.W., Ethics and evidence-based medicine: Fallibility and responsibility in clinical science. *JRSM*, 2003. **96**(5): p. 3-5.
10. Ibid.
11. Morabia, A., In defense of Pierre Louis who pioneered the

epidemiological approach to good medicine. *Journal of Clinical Epidemiology*, 2009. **62**(1): p. 1-4.

12. Wallenborn, W.M. George Washington's terminal illness: A modern medical analysis of the last illness and death of George Washington. 1999.

13. Crofton, J., The MRC randomized trial of streptomycin and its legacy: a view from the clinical front line. *Journal of the Royal Society of Medicine*, 2006. **99**(10): p. 531-534.

14. Sadowski, J., Non-partisan advice needed by congress., in Office of Technology Assessment Archive 2012.

15. (US), N.A.O.S., Council on Heath Care Technology, 1986 and 1987. 1987: National Academies.

16. Davidoff, F., B. Haynes, D. Sackett, and R. Smith, Evidence based medicine. *British Medical Journal*, 1995. **310**(6987): p. 1085.

CHAPTER 3

The Meaning of Significance and the Significance of Meaning

REPORTEDLY IN A letter to fellow physicist, Michael Faraday (1791-1867) asked of James Clerk Maxwell (1831-1879), "there is one thing that I would be glad to ask you. When a mathematician engaged in investigating physical actions and results has arrived at his own conclusions, may they not be expressed in common language as fully, clearly and definitely as in mathematical formulae?"(1)

I am uncertain as to how Maxwell responded, however, clinicians continue to ask that question, particularly those among us who were not formerly or rigorously trained in the language of research. Epidemiology is usually defined as the study of disease occurrence in populations. The primary units of concern, as Gary Friedman tells us, are groups of persons, not separate individuals, and the language of the discipline is biostatistics (2). In the next two chapters, an attempt will be made to explain the basics of this language to a lay or student audience. The goal will be to provide the reader with enough general information to understand how the results of clinical studies are reported, what criteria is used to determine if the results are significant within the discipline, what is implied by the term significance and more importantly, who should care other than the investigators, *i.e.* what is the clinical relevance or meaning for the rest of us.

There are two primary reasons why this is one of the shortest chapters. First my intention is to provide no more information for the reader not trained in statistics than is absolutely necessary to understand the strength or weaknesses, from a statistical standpoint, of the studies that we will discuss in subsequent chapters. Equally important, as a non-statistician, I don't want to try to explain more than I understand.

The main point or focus of this chapter will be to describe how researchers set out to prove that the difference that they have encountered in the results is due to an actual treatment effect and not due to chance. For example, if scientists are studying the efficacy (or effectiveness) of a drug for hypertension or diabetes and the drug is being compared to a placebo (a chemically or physiological inert substance, *i.e.* a "sugar pill"), they want to assess whether the drug's apparent efficacy does not represent some mere chance, or random, occurrence. The test, which is conducted to demonstrate genuine efficacy, is the significance test. By convention, the 5% level is taken as the cut off point. In other words, if the probability or "P value" is said to be less than 5 percent (usually expressed as $P = < 0.05$), this translates as there is less than 5 in a hundred times that the positive result would occur due to chance. The presumption here is that there is a real, genuine difference between the drug and the placebo or between one drug and another. This is felt to give validity to the study, internal validity, if you will. Internal, because it does not say that the validity internal to the study will have any relevance or validity to those who were not involved in the study; it does not predict *external* validity. Another way of expressing this is to say that the clinical significance of the result is not determined because the internal validity has been established. Once again, as my patients occasionally asked, "yeah, doc, but what does it have to do with me?" Precisely! The researchers and those reading the study may infer that the study result is relevant to others because of how carefully the study was designed. If my patient is a 55-year-old overweight African-American man, with 2 years of college and a salary of $50,000 and there were similar patients represented in the study, then the implication is that the result found in the study may also apply to my patient. Since we cannot possibly study everyone, having the subjects be as representative as possible may be the best that can be accomplished. Also, this is where the "law of large numbers," comes into play; that is, the larger the sample size, the greater chance you have, theoretically, of approaching the truth of whatever you are trying to establish. Even more convincing, if several large studies are done with similar populations and similar results are found, this affords even greater confidence, especially if the treatment effects found are "statistically significant." However, it is still the responsibility of the clinician to review the results of these various studies and determine if the results suggest clinical significance in light of what he knows of the patient in front of him and what his experience has been with a large body of patients whom she has treated over the years. Only she can determine this, not the researchers, academics, or reviewers of multiple studies. In this, the clinical process, the researcher serves as an assistant; providing material, data for the clinician to review and determine where and to what extent it is to be used, not slavishly following as if it represents THE EVIDENCE passed down from on high.

When doctors are making their treatment recommendations, whether they are sitting across from the patient in the office; at the bedside in the hospital; or via the radio, television or Internet; they are doing so, at best, on the basis of various "studies." This is particularly true of the medical professional who claims to be practicing EBM. This book is geared, not toward the reader who is content with accepting whatever the doctor recommends because he or she went to medical school and "should know what they're talking about," rather, I am speaking primarily to the person who believes it is important to know why the recommendations are being made. It seems reasonable that, if one is going to suggest or agree to a treatment that has potential hazards, in terms of morbidity and mortality (getting sick or dying), may be expensive, and is potentially life-long, a reasonable person would want to make some sense of where the recommendation is coming from. Therefore the following is for those who care, perhaps a minority. The specific types of studies we are referring to are generally those designed to test the efficacy of a treatment, particularly as compared to no treatment or, alternatively, multiple treatments may be compared to determine which is the most effective. There are various ways of obtaining evidence for the efficacy of a particular treatment, a case report, which describes the experience with one patient, or a case series involving several more patients. The form of investigation, however, which is regarded by most in the medical research world as the strongest method of obtaining evidence, the so-called "gold standard," is the randomized clinical trial. A clinical trial is a method of investigation where the researchers don't merely take a group of people with similar characteristics (cohort) and follow them over time to determine if they develop a particular condition, e.g. following smokers over time to determine how many develop lung cancer. Rather, the clinical trial is a form of experiment, whereby an intervention is performed; a drug or other treatment is given to one group and no treatment or alternate treatments are given to the other group (s). By randomized, we don't mean to imply that the persons are chosen randomly from the general population. More often than not, they are volunteers who are selected from a hospital, clinic, HMO or other site and they have met a series of entry and exclusion criteria that has been set up by the researchers. Over the years, I have heard countless patients refuse participation in trials or new treatments saying, "I don't want to be a guinea pig." Volunteers for a trial, however, must provide informed consent, which includes an explanation of the known risks and available alternatives. They have the right to withdraw from the study at any time for any reason. If the study is "blinded" the individuals do not know to which group — treatment or control — they have been assigned. Also, they are not able to receive any form of compensation for any potential adverse effects. The term randomization suggests that any one individual has an equal probability of being assigned to either the treatment or the control group. Randomization is felt to be the hallmark of controlled clinical trials and is why they are deemed to be most reliable. The process ideally minimizes, if not eliminates, selection bias. In other words, it is a way of preventing more individuals with risk factors for a disease in question from being assigned to one group than another. For example, suppose you are trying to determine if one anti-hypertensive drug is more effective than another and due to inadequate randomization, the treatment group contains younger, slimmer persons who are more accustomed to exercise; you might then expect to see that the treatment group over time has lower numbers and conclude, incorrectly, that the drug is more effective than placebo.

The randomized clinical trial, while much admired, is not easily done for a number of reasons. It is time consuming, requiring several years in some cases. For larger trials involving thousands of participants, millions of dollars are required. Therefore, it follows that it is usually governmental agencies or pharmaceutical companies that have the funds to carry out such investigations. There are also certain issues that do not easily lend themselves to the trial format. For example trials involving diets are difficult, as one has to rely on participants recalling what they ate in the immediate and remote past. Since standardization in vitamins and herbal products, for example, is difficult, it would be a challenge to study these substances and attempt to compare their efficacy to that of pharmaceuticals. Whereas a drug is likely to contain one chemical which is relatively easy to isolate and test, the herb, on the other hand, is likely to contain various substances, all of which may contribute to its efficacy. Therefore, many of the recommendations regarding these non-standardized substances can be said to be essentially based upon anecdotal information. This is not to say that this information is without value.

As alluded to above, another important feature of the trial is "blindedness;" that is, a study is said to be a single blinded study if the participants do not know to which group they have been assigned; treatment or placebo. A double-blinded study is when neither the study patients nor the investigators know to which group the participants have been assigned. Therefore, according to current thinking in the medical research community, the strongest evidence is provided by the double-blinded, placebo controlled randomized clinical trial, involving large numbers of people and ideally duplicated by other investigators.

When the trial has been completed and the results are to be analyzed, various statistical tests are used. The purpose of a statistical test is to determine whether some hypothesis (proposed explanation) is extremely unlikely given the observed data. This next point is not the easiest to understand but I will give it a try. The investigator, or specifically the statistician, starts with the premise that, if for example the efficacy of 2 treatments are being studied, that there is no difference between the treatments. This is called the "null hypothesis," *i.e.* there is no difference. Whether or not there is thought to be a difference in the treatments is expressed in the form of the "p" value. Although, admittedly arbitrary, the p value of 5%, as noted above, is almost universally regarded as the cut-off level for statistical significance. A statistically significant difference is one that cannot be accounted for by chance alone. Stay with me, now. Another way of saying this is, if the p value is determined to be less than 5%, then whatever difference is noted between the treatments is likely due to a REAL difference in the treatments and not chance alone (as in the flip of a coin). So when a researcher reports a finding as being statistically significant, they're implying that a genuine difference in treatments is suggested. It should be pointed out, however, that the reverse or converse is not necessarily the case, *i.e.* if a difference is found not to be statistically significant, it doesn't follow that this can be explained by chance alone.

There are a number of factors that can result in a difference being not statistically significant, but first a word about sampling error. The process of sampling is inherently flawed. It is based on the basic "principle that if many random samples are obtained, rates calculated from the data in those samples *on the average* (italics mine) will be the same as the rate of the original population" (3). Therefore, each sample could have either a lower or higher rate than the original population and since the sample is only accurate, on average, any individual sample is said to have a fundamental sampling error. If the sample size is small, the degree of sampling error can be large and this often leads to a non-significant test even if the observed difference is caused by a *real* treatment effect. There is said to be no reliable way to determine if a non-significant difference is due to the small sample size or because the null hypothesis ("there is no difference") is correct. This is why statisticians use mathematical equations before the study is begun to determine how many participants need to be involved in order to observe a real treatment effect, if one truly exists. This is referred to as the "power" of a study, *i.e.* is the sample size large enough, and is the study adequately powered to observe a treatment effect. Therefore, when medical types quote from studies and assert that the results are statistically significant they are describing the tidiness of the study; it's internal validity and this is the reason why a result that is not statistically significant should, at best, be regarded as inconclusive rather than an inference of no treatment effect. I realize that this may all sound needlessly confusing but it is important for those among us who are giving or being given recommendations and affected by medical policy and who wish to be more than sheep, to at least begin to understand what these people are talking about. Although numbers and graphs can often be intimidating, there is a very useful message which is given by Darrell Huff in a book published close to sixty years ago but still timely, *How To Lie With Statistics*, "despite its mathematical base, statistics is as much an art as it is a science. A great many manipulations and even distortions are possible within the bounds of propriety. Often the statistician must choose among methods, a subjective process and find the one that he will use to represent the *facts* (italics mine)" (4).

When the various statistical criteria have been met, the study can be said to demonstrate internal validity. Indeed but "what does that have to do with me, doc?" which brings us to the next section.

References Cited

1. Kline, M., *Mathematics and the Search for Knowledge.* New York: Oxford University Press, 1985. p.145.
2. Friedman, G.D., *Primer of Epidemiology.* New York: McGraw-Hill Book. 1994. p.1.
3. Riegelman, R.K. and R.P. Hirsch, *Studying a Study and Testing a Test.* Philadelphia: Lippincott Williams & Wilkins, 2005. p.193.
4. Huff, D., *How to Lie with Statistics.* New York: Norton, 1982. p.122.

CHAPTER 4

Extrapolation — The Leap of Faith

IN MATHEMATICS, IT is said that extrapolation is the process of constructing new data points outside a discrete set of known data points. In statistics, specifically, to extrapolate is to draw conclusions about something beyond the range of the data. Using a hypothetical example, if you study 10, 100, 1000 or more individuals, analyze the results and, based upon the results found in the sample, attempt to make inferences about what is true in the larger population, who were not involved in the study, then you are attempting to extrapolate. On some level, this is done all the time and is understandable. It is not possible to study everyone, except in a census if everyone is counted; therefore, the best we can hope for is a sample, however large or small. The hope is that the sample will be as representative of the general population as possible and that, even conceding individual variability, we can, nonetheless, make assumptions that have relevance to a larger group than the study sample. Granted, this involves a lot of assuming, hoping and inferring, but it is the best we can do. If we don't extrapolate, then the researcher remains confined to their own universe of data, which may be interesting, but is about individuals who may have little to do with the rest of us. Sometimes, in fact, this is the reality of what is done; however, no one wants to concede that. For example our concept of "normal bone density" was originally based upon 1994 WHO (World Health Organization) recommendations for white women. There have been several studies since the initial WHO guidelines, most recently one published in the *New England Journal of Medicine* in January of 2012 (1), but even there the researchers acknowledged that the study population was limited to women 67 years and older, 99 percent of whom were white. Despite such limitations we are expected to, unapologetically, make recommendations to all, at least middle-aged and elderly women in this country based upon these studies.

In close to 30 years of clinical medicine, I have heard on countless occasions that one or another high-blood pressure medicines is either particularly effective or ineffective in African-Americans, for example. More often than not, I find little correlation in my patient population or in those of several other colleagues. Is it that our patient base is so different than that of other physicians? Not necessarily. More likely it's just that our patients were not involved in the studies upon which the recommendations were made. They represent a different data set, if you will. Navigating through a number of epidemiology and statistics texts, one is struck with the degree of confidence the authors express in the validity of various statistical tests and the ability to extrapolate. Often what one is made aware of are the futile attempts to predict individual human behavior via reduction to mathematical formulae. Perhaps this criticism may be dismissed as that of a person who has spent approximately 40 years between social work and clinical medicine, having learned a few things about human behavior, but still knowing little about mathematics, and therefore, often failing to appreciate the connection. The gist of my argument is that it is highly questionable as to how confidently one can use data obtained in a sampled population and apply the data to the unsampled population. It would appear that this presumption can be neatly made only within the context of a

31

mathematical equation. It is not for the researcher to extrapolate. It is understandable that the investigator is in no position to address issues of interest to any given doctor or community. It, therefore, has to be up to the individual health care professional to make sense of the data provided, apply it where applicable and discard it when irrelevant.

The more carefully one selects the sample, the more representative it is likely to be of the general population. If the sample reflects the general population in terms of age, gender, socio-economic status, ethnicity, and educational level, then we are likely to be more confident in our extrapolation. Even if the investigators are extraordinarily diligent in their selection and control of the various factors listed above, there will still be individual variables that cannot be accounted for and controlled. It is well known that even identical twins (formed from the same fertilized egg) can react differently to environmental or pharmacological stimuli (2, 3). The objective of this apparent departure is to illustrate, once again, the hazards of extrapolation even under the best of circumstances and where the subjects are even genetically identical. There is a tendency of the devotees of a discipline to become so enamored as to get lost in the elegance of their formulations. Our primary concern, however, as clinicians is to understand how our patients will be best served by a certain recommendation and how to explain it in language they can understand. What the patient then does with that information, perhaps listening inattentively and saying, "whatever you say, doc," is beyond our control. This attempt to extrapolate on the part of investigators and to accept, as valid, such attempts, exemplifies a tendency alluded to in the chapter on EBM; it is as if the methodologists suffer from an inherent sense of inferiority. Because of the success of physical science, many of those doing clinical (people) research seek to don the mantle of scientific respectability. Once again, we are dealing with human behavior, using samples of a population, usually made up of volunteers, who may or may not be representative of a limited population and attempting to make inferences about individuals who were not studied. There are no verifiable laws that have been duplicated, that are being generated, and therefore only the form, the method, is scientific.

Too often, the methodology is based upon unjustified assumptions. The sample is defined as the data that were collected and the population is the data which would have been collected if you had conducted the study "an infinite" number of times. It is often said that learning novel meanings for commonly used words and concepts is part of the inherent difficulty of understanding statistics. For example, a core concept of statistics is the "normal population." This is an assumption that researchers, or more specifically statisticians, make about the population from which the sample is selected. They assume that the sample follows a special distribution known as the bell-shaped or normal distribution. In a normal distribution, very large or very small values are rare, while average values are more common. If we were to construct a normal distribution of the heights of adult males within a given community (Figure 1), for example, we would likely find that most of the men would be found toward the center of the curve, with the very short and very tall individuals at either tail end. This distribution is called "normal" or the standard against which other distributions may be compared. In general, once you assume that the population follows a normal distribution, statistical tests then allow you to make inferences, or extrapolate, about that population.

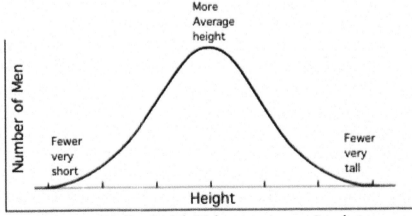

Figure 1. Heights of Adult Males in an Average Population.

Another presumptuous method used by statisticians to validate extrapolation is a process known as resampling. This is more likely to be performed in laboratory experiments but is also seen in clinical research. A practical problem is that statistical inferences can only apply to the population from which the sample was derived and you want to extend the inferences beyond the collected data. Therefore you can make conclusions about what "would" happen, *i.e.* hypothetically, if you repeated the study several more times. A practical way of accomplishing this is through the use of computer-generated programs, with methods that have intriguing names such as Bootstrap, Jackknife and Monte Carlo simulations, for example. Hopefully you can appreciate that the value of going through this list of required assumptions is to further illustrate the hazards of extrapolation in people research. We are justified in being at least skeptical of drawing conclusions from information gathered under questionable circumstances (the unknown) and summarily applying it to our patients (the known). We need not apologize for not fully understanding this discipline, for many of the manipulations are inexplicable and essentially faith-based. This is what I alluded to earlier when it was suggested that what we don't understand, we tend to revere.

The media, in 20 second sound bytes, report the findings in these studies; often creating fear and apprehension, making certain that you tune in at 11 to get all of the "details" which can be provided in 90 seconds; coffee, alcohol, vitamin supplements are good… no, they're bad.

To summarize where we are at this point; to extrapolate from a sample to the larger population, we want to infer that the mean, or central tendency, results found in the sample, are applicable to the general population. As a reminder, the mean is the average where you add up all the numbers in a sample and then divide by the total of the numbers. So : 15+20+10+7+12+ = 64/5 = 12.8 (mean). If a sample is small and variable, the sample mean may be quite far from the population mean. If your sample is large with little variability (often called "scatter") the sample mean will "more likely" be closer to the population mean. Statistical calculations use sample mean and scatter to generate something called a "confidence interval." Statisticians can calculate intervals for any degree of confidence, but 95% intervals are most commonly used. The following example will illustrate how these intervals are reported and hopefully clarify what must appear as offering greater confusion than it is worth: If two drugs, A and B for weight loss are studied and drug A is found to be more effective, it may be said that the confidence interval (CI) at the 95 percent level reveals a mean weight loss of 10–15 pounds during the course of the study. Translation: if this study were repeated 100 times, we can say that 95 percent of the time the mean weight loss with drug A would be somewhere between 10–15 pounds. The results appear more convincing the narrower the intervals are. For example, if the 95% level revealed an interval of between 5–20 pounds, this would be considered a weaker finding than the preceding because in the latter case the mean is "all over the place" some subjects losing as little as five pounds and some as much as 20 pounds. With Drug A, there appears to be a more predictable degree of weight lost (10–15 pounds). Again, "if you accept the assumptions," there is a 95% chance that the interval that was calculated includes the true difference between population means. We are told that in mathematics, extrapolation doesn't always work, and it also gets worse as you extrapolate further from your known data. Sometimes, however, because of the difficulty, if not impossibility, of obtaining good, reliable data in large populations, extrapolation is the best we can achieve, but it is always to be regarded with considerable skepticism.

References Cited

1. Gourlay, M.L., J.P. Fine, J.S. Preisser, R.C. May, C. Li, L.-Y. Lui, D.F. Ransohoff, J.A. Cauley, and K.E. Ensrud, Bone-density

testing interval and transition to osteoporosis in older women. *New England Journal of Medicine*, 2012. **366**(3): p. 225-233.

2. Rahmioğlu, N. and K.R. Ahmadi, Classical twin design in modern pharmacogenomics studies. *Pharmacogenomics*, 2010. **11**(2): p. 215-226.

3. Bell, J.T. and T.D. Spector, A twin approach to unraveling epigenetics. *Trends in Genetics*, 2011. **27**(3): p. 116-125.

CHAPTER 5

Prostate Cancer Screening

THE PROSTATE GLAND is usually described as a walnut-sized organ, weighing approximately 1 ounce, located just below the bladder and pressing up against the front of the rectum . During the male orgasm, it produces a fluid that is a constituent of semen, the purpose of which is to protect and nourish the sperm during its journey to fertilize (or not) the ovum in the female uterus. Infection or inflammation of the prostate (prostatitis) can occur in any age group, the causes of which are often uncertain. It is said to be the most common reason for which men under 50 years in the United States visit the office of a urologist. The prostate condition that is of greater public health significance, however, and which is the subject of this chapter, is prostate cancer. To give a sense of how great a public health problem is posed by prostate cancer, a brief rehashing of well-publicized numbers is probably in order. According to the American Cancer Society's 2010 estimates, there are 217,730 new cases of the cancer each year, accounting for 32,000 deaths (1). Except for skin cancer, it is the most common form of cancer found in American men and it is the second leading cause of cancer death behind lung cancer.

Risk factors for prostate cancer include age, race and heredity.

While it is certainly not unheard of to have the disease diagnosed in the forties, it is primarily a disease of older men. Although anecdotal, in my 28 years of general internal medicine practice, having had numerous men diagnosed with prostate cancer, overwhelmingly, they were in their sixties and older. As to why older men are more likely to develop prostate cancer, like so many things in medicine, this is a matter of debate. There are a number of hypotheses, which contend that the hormonal changes of aging place older men at risk, however, none of the arguments are consistent and convincing and therefore not too useful to debate in a book geared toward a general or student audience. Concerning the role of race, it is acknowledged that African-American men have the world's highest incidence of prostate cancer — one third higher than that of white men. Whenever negative statistics are reported with respect to black men, the reasons are often attributed to lifestyle or socioeconomic factors. In the past, it was presumed that African-American men were more likely to develop prostate cancer due to poverty, decreased access to medical care with delayed diagnosis and follow-up and poor (*i.e.* high-saturated fat) diet. Interestingly, however, in December of 2000, a group of Harvard researchers published the results of a 10-year study that tracked the development of prostate cancer within a group of 45,000 male health professionals including doctors, pharmacists and optometrists (2). African-Americans in the study were still more than twice as likely to develop prostate cancer, yet all of the men had similar incomes and educational backgrounds, suggesting that they had similar diets and were equally as likely to receive regular medical evaluations. The Harvard researchers did detect a genetic difference among the black men in the study. Proteins on the prostate cells known as androgen receptors were more likely to exhibit a slight alteration. Androgen receptors bind to hormones such as testosterone, which was felt by some in the medical community dating back to the 1940s, to promote the growth of prostate cancer (3). In the interest of full disclosure, this is another area of great controversy.

Boston Urologist, Abraham Morgantaler, in his 2009 book, *Testosterone For Life*, devotes a chapter to essentially refuting the long held claim that testosterone promotes prostate cancer growth (4). Therefore, this variation in androgen receptors may not explain the higher prostate cancer rates in black men.

In a 2004 paper Robin Vollmer (5) discussed the linkage between race and PSA level. He noted that, in general, the level of PSA reflects the amount of tumor present. He found that black men produced higher levels of PSA for any given amount of tumor compared to whites and that this could indicate differences in outcome. He suggests that differences in the development of blood vessels (angiogenesis) may partially explain these racial differences. Angiogenesis, is important because it enables the tumor to thrive and spread elsewhere in the body. Furthermore, this is important because, not only are black men more likely to develop prostate cancer, but they are also 2 to 3 times more likely to die from it. The bottom line, however, is that this is another in a series of proposals that await confirmation. In 2003, University of Iowa urology professor, Richard Williams, revealed some numbers, revised in 2006, that if three relatives have prostate cancer, you are 10 times more likely to develop the disease (6). Further, if your father or brother have prostate cancer, you are 2 to 3 times more likely to develop it. So there is consensus as to the risk factors — age, race and heredity, but the precise reasons are unknown. With all of this gloom and uncertainty, there appears to be some relatively good news. Compared to most cancers, prostate cancer tends to grow very slowly and it could be several decades from the time that the initial abnormal changes can be seen microscopically in prostate tissue, and when symptoms develop. As an aside, the symptoms of prostate cancer are nonspecific and may include the following: frequent urination, inability to urinate, difficulty in starting or stopping the stream of urination, weak or interrupted flow of urine, and/or pain or burning on urination. These symptoms are said to be nonspecific because a man can have any of these complaints and not have cancer. More often than not, these symptoms are found in those with a benign (non-cancerous) enlargement of the prostate. Commonly, men with prostate cancer will not have any symptoms.

So these characteristics of prostate cancer; that it tends to be very slow growing and is frequently without symptoms, theoretically at least, makes it a good candidate for screening. Screening is usually defined as the application of tests, procedures or examinations in an attempt to identify unrecognized disease. For the venture to be successful, the tests should be rapidly applied, relatively inexpensive, minimally invasive and well tolerated by the patient. This is one of the reasons why mass colon cancer screening with sigmoidoscopy is not feasible; the expense and technical expertise required, preparation needed prior to testing, time it takes to perform the procedure and the public perception of unpleasantness is too great. Screening is a strategy designed to sort out those seemingly well persons who have a disease from those who do not have the disease. The screening test is not meant to give a definitive diagnosis. If a person tests positive, they still need to follow up with a health professional for further workup and definitive testing and treatment when indicated. Positive tests are merely suggestive that a problem may exist. Screening may be conducted as part of an epidemiological survey (remember epidemiology is the study of disease occurrence in human populations) to determine the natural history or prevalence of a condition of public health importance. At this point a couple of definitions are in order: prevalence is a measure of how many cases of a disease *currently* exist whereas incidence is the number of *new* cases of a disease. One of the most well known epidemiological surveys, for example, is the Framingham Study of Coronary Heart Disease, which has been ongoing since 1948. Screenings also may be conducted to detect or prevent a contagious disease or to protect those at risk for a disease. A smaller example is the Tb screening which I was a part of in a 900-bed shelter for homeless men in 1993 (7). Certain groups at high risk for a certain disease can be identified on the basis of race, age, gender or socioeconomic status. Screening of such groups will have a higher yield than surveying an unselected population. Therefore, the survey should be aimed at a population with a presumed higher prevalence of the disease of interest. In 1993, we therefore assumed that we would obtain a higher yield by screening the homeless population than, for example, Columbia University students a few blocks away.

I listed a few characteristics above for a good screening test; now a word about which diseases particularly lend themselves to screening. The disease should be relatively common in the population, such as diabetes, hypertension (high blood pressure), or heart disease. The condition should be of great public health importance with significant morbidity and mortality (leading to sickness and/or death). We should be able to identify the disease or the suggestion of it relatively easily with the use of a good screening test. It also is important that the disease in question have a long lead-time. Lead-time is defined as the interval between the time the condition is detected through screening and the time it would normally have been detected by the reporting of symptoms or signs. Therefore conditions such diabetes, hypertension, prostate and breast cancer generally have long lead times, *i.e.* several years may pass between being able to detect evidence of it through screening and the time at which symptoms or overt signs of it or its consequences may develop. Finally, the disease for which we are screening should have a treatment or cure. It makes little sense to screen for a condition about which we can do nothing. What is the value of detecting a disease, early in the process that has no cure, only to leave the patient fearful, apprehensive and miserable for the rest of their life? The focus of this chapter, prostate cancer, would seem to be a particularly apt condition for screening. It is relatively common in the general population, as indicated by the American Cancer Society numbers quoted in the beginning. It is said that there are some 2 million men in this country who have been diagnosed with prostate cancer at some time in their life. It is of public health importance, accounting for approximately 32,000 deaths annually. The PSA test, which if it has a high enough number can suggest that "there is a problem with the prostate," is easy to do. (More about the test later). Lead-time is generally quite long, from several years to possibly decades.

Before discussing the PSA test, a few additional words are in order concerning the characteristics desired in a screening test. The test should have a high validity. Important determinants of validity are sensitivity and specificity. Sensitivity means how accurately the test is able to truly identify those persons who are positive; *i.e.* of those with a "positive" test, how many truly have the disease. If the test is positive and the person does not have the disease, then it is a false positive. If there are too many false positives, then the test is said to have low, or poor sensitivity. Specificity means how accurately the test identifies those persons who are truly negative; *i.e.* of those with a "negative" test, how many do not have the disease. If a person has a negative test, but ultimately is shown to have the disease — that represents a false negative. Too many false negatives makes for a test of poor or low specificity. The screening test should be reliable; accurate results can be duplicated across a large population. The test should be able to produce a high yield; identify large numbers who are truly positive or negative. How well does the PSA test fulfill the foregoing criteria?

PSA (Prostate Specific Antigen) is a protein that is made by cells within the prostate gland and is said to be the substance that accounts for the liquid quality of semen. Most of the PSA leaves the body with the semen, but some is retained and enters the blood. As men become older, the prostate gland enlarges, almost inevitably. During my training the rule of thumb used to be that by age 80, approximately 80 percent of men would have an enlarged prostate. As it becomes larger, more PSA is produced, therefore it is presumed that older men will have higher values, without necessarily having any indication of cancer. In America, the upper limit of normal is 4.0, but in the United

Kingdom and other countries in Europe, 3.0 is generally accepted as the upper limit. Recognizing that PSA production tends to increase with age, some researchers and clinicians are actually using what is called age-specific PSA levels to determine what is an acceptable level. Age-specific upper limits for PSA may be as follows: age 40–49 is 2.5, 50–59 is 3.5, 60–69 is 4.5, 70–79 is 6.5 (8). The use of age-specific PSA levels for the diagnosis of prostate cancer is, as you might expect, controversial. Not all studies have agreed that using age-specific levels are better than simply using the cutoff level of 4.0 across all age groups.

Although the primary purpose for drawing PSA blood levels is to look for early evidence of cancer; most elevations are not caused by cancer. Other causes of elevated PSA include benign prostate enlargement, prostatitis, or recent sexual activity. An elevated PSA, therefore, only suggests that there is "an issue" with the prostate, which may or may not be cancer. Approximately 80 percent of the time an elevated PSA does not indicate cancer (9). Again, there was a rule of thumb, now regarded as outmoded, that if the initial PSA is 10 or greater, it is far more likely to represent cancer. This adage is becoming passé, probably because since the PSA test became commonly used in the 1980s, it is now unusual to find a man over 40 who has not had the test done. A significant number of men over the age of 50 are accustomed to having the test done periodically; at least annually, therefore, a workup and treatment will likely be done long before a man's level will get to 10. In the last 10 years, most of the men who were diagnosed with prostate cancer in my practice had levels less than 10 and as low as 5.8 (in their early 60s). There is no level of PSA that effectively rules out the possibility of cancer. Although quite uncommon, there have been cases of cancer reported with PSA levels of less than 4.0 (10). At the other extreme, I have treated several men over the years with PSA levels in the range of 10–40, but who had symptoms or signs of prostatitis (urinary frequency, painful urination, tender prostate on exam), were treated with antibiotics and, within days to weeks, their PSA levels returned to normal. It has always been apparent to me, that if our primary concern and reason for testing PSA level is cancer, then the test is not at all specific and has questionable sensitivity. There is literature that supports this.

Several studies (11-13) demonstrate that if a man has prostate cancer and a PSA level is drawn, approximately 86% of the time the test will be abnormal (when 4.0 is selected as the upper limit of normal). This is an indication of the test's sensitivity, meaning the percentage of time that those with disease are correctly identified. This level is considered "pretty good." The specificity of the test; however, how accurately we identify with a negative test those who do not have the disease, is only 34 percent. So the test is good for identifying "issues" with the prostate, but not necessarily cancer, but that is our main concern. Just as there are a number of benign causes for elevated PSA, prostate cancer may be present with presumably "normal" levels, as alluded to above. The fact that there is a risk of prostate cancer at all levels of PSA was made clear in a 2004 study published in the *New England Journal of Medicine* (14) where prostate cancer was shown to occur at very low PSA levels (Table 1).

Table 1. Relationship of PSA level with the Prevalence of Prostate Cancer		
PSA Level	Number of Men Tested	Men with Prostate Cancer
≤0.5 ng/mL	486	32
0.6–1.0 ng/mL	791	80
1.1–2.0 ng/mL	998	170
2.1–3.0 ng/mL	482	115
3.1-4.0 ng/mL	193	52

At least one message here is that there is always risk; we can minimize but not eliminate it and this is true with medicine and, in general, life. Above, we said that the overall sensitivity of the test was 86 percent which is "pretty good," that means that 14 percent of the time a man with a normal level (here less than 4.0) will actually have cancer. This is called a false negative. So we can improve the 86 percent sensitivity by lowering the cutoff value of what is considered the upper limit of normal, but the downside is to increase the number of false positives. This will lead to more biopsies of the prostate for men who do not have cancer. Prostate biopsy is not brain or heart surgery, but there are some risks; bleeding and infection; some adverse or at least annoying consequences; mild to moderate discomfort, hours of blood in the urine following the procedure and days of blood in the semen (should one be in the mood to produce semen during this period).

The total PSA test has certain limitations and this has led to the recommendation of assessments that are more precise, such as measuring free PSA. Some of the PSA is bound to other proteins — complexed PSA — and some remains unbound — free PSA. Most of the time it is the total PSA — complexed plus free — that is measured, but increasingly doctors are distinguishing between the free and complexed component because of presumed greater accuracy or specificity for assessing the likelihood of cancer. Some recommend measuring the complexed (cPSA) as it is deemed more predictive of cancer and would lead to fewer false diagnoses and unnecessary biopsies. These limitations in sensitivity and specificity of the PSA test have resulted in approximately 1 million biopsies being performed in this country annually (15). For every 4 men who undergo the biopsy, only one will prove to have cancer (16). This has led to even greater efforts to find a more specific test such as a genetic marker for prostate cancer which is unique to the individual, specific, less invasive and easy to perform. There is such a test, the so-called PCA3, which is a genetic marker that is found in the urine. Within the lab, the test has been found to be reliable and accurate, however, there are still a number of unresolved issues that will be addressed in further clinical research trials before the test becomes available.

The goal of screening is to detect a disease early enough in its course to either cure it or significantly decrease mortality; that is to increase the length of time that one can live with the disease if a cure is not possible. Therefore the basic question requiring an answer is whether, by screening with the PSA test, we are prolonging the life of the man in whom cancer is detected because the treatments available are more effective than not treating ("watchful waiting"). Over the years several studies have been conducted to answer this question. Following is a brief description of the results of some of these larger studies.

The European Randomized Study of Screening for Prostate Cancer (ERSPC) (17) was designed in the early 1990s primarily to determine the death rate from prostate cancer. There were 182,160 participants between the ages of 50–74 recruited from multiple centers in seven European countries. The men were randomly assigned to a group of 82,816 who were offered PSA screening an average of once every 4 years and a control group of 99,184 who did not receive screening. Most of the centers used a PSA cutoff of 3.0 (ng/milliliter) as an indication for biopsy to definitely make the diagnosis. Of all the men who underwent biopsy for an elevated PSA, 76 percent of them were determined *not* to have cancer, *i.e.* they had "false positive" PSA tests. Overall, they detected 5990 prostate cancers in the screening group and 4307 in the control group. As of 2006, with an average follow-up period of 9 years, there were 214 prostate cancer deaths in the screening group and 326 in the control group. The researchers concluded that PSA screening reduced the rate of death from prostate cancer by 20 percent but was associated with a high risk of over diagnosis, which was defined as a positive diagnosis in men who would not have had clinical symptoms during their lifetime. These are examples of the men who would have likely died *with* rather than *from* prostate cancer. This rate of over diagnosis in the above study was estimated to be as high as 50 percent. In chapter 4 we spoke about the risks involved in extrapolating beyond the limits of any given study. Such risks may also be apparent in this study.

The American-based Prostate, Lung, Colorectal and Ovarian (PLCO) trial was conducted almost simultaneously with the ERSPC (18). From 1993–2001, over 75,000 men between the ages of 55–74 were enrolled at 10 different centers throughout the United States. The participants were assigned to one of two groups; one who received annual PSA and digital rectal screening and the control group that did not. After 7 years, there were 50 deaths attributed to prostate cancer in the screening group and 44 in the control group; the difference was neither statistically nor clinically significant. After 10 years, there were 92 prostate cancer deaths in the screening group and 82 in the control group. The researchers concluded that after 7–10 years, the rate of prostate cancer deaths was very low and did not differ significantly between the two groups. Therefore in this population of greater than 75,000, PSA and digital rectal screening did not affect mortality from cancer or other causes. This study has been criticized on several grounds. First, it used a PSA cutoff of 4.0, regarded by many as outdated. The study permitted the enrollment of a large percentage of men who had undergone previous prostate screening in the 2 to 3 years prior to the enrollment and consequently were very likely at lower risk. The control group included men who also underwent screening, thereby contaminating the results. The average follow-up was 5–6 years for men with cancers, which is not considered long enough for a cancer with relatively favorable prognosis; therefore the time period was too short to expect metastases or death.

There are three more clinical trials of note — one completed and two which are still on-going — which attempt to compare the effects of surgical intervention (removal of the entire prostate) versus watchful waiting in men with early, localized cancer (19-21). From 1989–1999, 695 men with early-stage cancer from 14 hospitals in 3 Scandinavian countries were enrolled in a trial. The average age of the men was 64.7 years and they were assigned either to the watchful waiting or radical prostatectomy group. The results of the trial after 8.2 years of follow-up were published in *The New England Journal of Medicine* (22).

1. 83 men in the surgery group and 106 in the watchful waiting group died.

2. In 30 of the 347 men assigned to the surgery and 50 of the 348 men assigned to watchful waiting, death was due to prostate cancer.

3. In terms of local progression and distant metastases, there was a several-fold percentage point increase of death in the watchful waiting group.

The researchers concluded that, compared to watchful waiting, radical prostatectomy reduces prostate cancer death and overall mortality and the risks of metastases and local progression. The absolute reduction in the risk of death after 10 years is small, but the reduction in the risks of metastases and local tumor progression are substantial. The lesson that some have taken from this single study is that radical surgery is a better approach than watchful waiting particularly for younger men; 65 or younger who, in the absence of other illnesses have a reasonable life expectancy of 10 to 15 years.

The generalizability of these findings is questionable. These were Scandinavian men who were initially diagnosed with prostate cancer because they had abnormal rectal examinations. In comparison, the majority of men diagnosed in the United States and Europe have a normal exam and an elevated PSA at the time of their diagnosis. There are two recent studies that attempted to enroll a more representative sample of men with early stage cancer.

The Prostate Cancer Intervention Versus Observation Trial (PIVOT) (23) was initiated in 1994 and is designed to determine whether radical surgery or watchful waiting provides greater length and quality of life for men with localized cancer. It is being conducted by the Department of Veteran Affairs and The National Cancer Institute. It involves multiple centers and although over 13,000 men were screened and over 5,000 met the initial eligibility criteria, only

731 agreed to participate. The average age of the participants is 67 and, of note, nearly one-third of the men are African-American (a group, as mentioned earlier, has the highest rate and poorest prognosis of prostate cancer in the world). After 12 years of follow – up, it was found that radical surgery did not significantly reduce prostate -cancer nor all cause mortality.

The Prostate Testing for Cancer and Treatment Trial (PROTECT-T) (24) was initiated in 2001 and the anticipated completion date is December of 2015. The study enrolled over 94,000 men in nine cities in the United Kingdom. Men with a PSA of 3 or higher were offered biopsies. The age, PSA, stage and grade at diagnosis of the participants with cancer were compared with information from unscreened prostate cancer patients, aged 50–69 from a United Kingdom cancer registry. As of 2012, the preliminary results are as follows:

1. A total of 50 percent of all of those who were invited agreed to participate.
2. Of those 94,000 men, 8,800 had an elevated PSA.
3. 2,022 men with an elevated PSA had prostate cancer by biopsy.
4. 239 men had locally advanced or metastatic disease. All other patients had localized disease.

This study was designed to evaluate the outcomes of three different approaches; surgery, radiation or "active monitoring." After 10 years, it was found that death from prostate cancer was low irrespective of the approach used.

So what are we to do in light of the studies completed thus far. As clinicians, we are to do, hopefully, what the sensible among us have always done. We need to continue to have one-on-one, frank conversations with our patients. If they wish to know, we need to inform them of the controversies, the questions that still linger. We need to determine what their individual risks may be (are they African-American, do they have a family history of prostate cancer?). We need to inform patients of the potential adverse effects of treatment and try to assess if the risks of treatment, versus watchful waiting, while certainly not inevitable, are tolerable. Many patients will defer to the provider, stating, "Doc, what do you think I should do?" However unsatisfying it may be for the individual patient, we must continue to stress the point that risks, and potential consequences are the patient's and so must be the burden of decision making. Our role as caregivers, particularly in an outpatient, non-emergency setting, is to provide as much information as is necessary so that whatever decision made is an informed one.

When I was in medical training during the late 1970s and early 1980s, we were taught that a man was likely to die with prostate cancer rather than because of it. This belief was based upon the fact that autopsies of several men in their 80s and older revealed evidence of prostate cancer, which was not known to the patient or his family and which did not appear to have any effect on the quality of his life. We were taught that most men in their 70s with a diagnosis of prostate cancer just required "watchful waiting," monitoring but no treatment. In official (urological) circles, watchful waiting appears to be a thing of the past. I have had several patients in their 80s during the past 10 years who were being treated for prostate cancer by their urologists (I know, anecdotal). Throughout contemporary American medicine, watchful waiting is increasingly regarded as inappropriate, passé. In this country, particularly, the feeling in medicine is "don't just stand there, do something!" Failure to intervene, whether it be in the personal lives of its citizens or in medicine, is usually out of the question, virtually un-American.

References Cited

1. Jemal, A., R. Siegel, J. Xu, and E. Ward, Cancer statistics, 2010. *CA: A Cancer Journal for Clinicians*, 2010. **60**(5): p. 277-300.

2. Platz, E.A., E.B. Rimm, W.C. Willett, P.W. Kantoff, and E. Giovannucci, Racial variation in prostate cancer incidence and in hormonal system markers among male health professionals. *Journal of the National Cancer Institute*, 2000. **92**(24): p. 2009-2017.

3. Huggins, C., R. Stevens, and C.V. Hodges, Studies on prostatic cancer II. The effects of castration on advanced carcinoma of the prostate gland. *Archives of Surgery*, 1941. **43**(2): p. 209-223.

4. Morgantaler, A., *Testosterone for Life: Recharge Your Vitality, Sex Drive, Muscle Mass & Overall Health!* New York: McGraw-Hill, 2009.

5. Vollmer, R.T. Race and the linkage between serum prostate-specific antigen and prostate cancer : A study of American veterans. *Am. J. Clin. Pathol.* 2004. **122**:.p. 338-344.

6. Williams, R. *Prostate cancer is the most common cancer in men.* 2006 [cited 2013 March 9] Available from: http://www.uihealthcare.org/2column.aspx?id=236746.

7. Paul, E.A., S.M. Lebowitz, R.E. Moore, C.W. Hoven, B.A. Bennett, and A. Chen, Nemesis revisited: tuberculosis infection in a New York City men's shelter. *American Journal of Public Health*, 1993. **83**(12): p. 1743-1745.

8. Mausner, J.S. and A.K. Bahn, *Epidemiology: An Introductory Text.* Philadelphia: Saunders, 1985.

9. Oesterling, J.E. and C.G. Chute, Serum Prostate-Specific Antigen in Community-Based Population. *Journal American Medical Association*, 1993. **270**: p. 860-864.

10. Hoffman, R.M., F.D. Gilliland, M. Adams-Cameron, W.C. Hunt, and C.R. Key, Prostate-specific antigen testing accuracy in community practice. *BMC Family Practice*, 2002. **3**(1): p. 19.

11. Thompson, I.M., D.P. Ankerst, C. Chi, M.S. Lucia, P.J. Goodman,

J.J. Crowley, H.L. Parnes, and C.A. Coltman Jr, Operating characteristics of prostate-specific antigen in men with an initial PSA level of 3.0 ng/ml or lower. *JAMA*, 2005. **294**(1): p. 66-70.

12. Thompson, I.M., D.K. Pauler, P.J. Goodman, C.M. Tangen, M.S. Lucia, H.L. Parnes, L.M. Minasian, L.G. Ford, S.M. Lippman, and E.D. Crawford, Prevalence of prostate cancer among men with a prostate-specific antigen level≤ 4.0 ng per milliliter. *New England Journal of Medicine*, 2004. **350**(22): p. 2239-2246.

13. Mettlin, C., P.J. Littrup, R.A. Kane, G.P. Murphy, F. Lee, A. Chesley, R. Badalament, and F.K. Mostofi, Relative sensitivity and specificity of serum prostate specific antigen (PSA) level compared with age-referenced PSA, PSA density, and PSA change. *Cancer*, 1994. **74**(5): p. 1615-1620.

14. Thompson, *et al. New England Journal of Medicine*, 2004. **350**(22): p. 2239-2246.

15. Irwin, K. Prostate cancer now detectable using imaging-guided biopsy, UCLA study shows. UCLA Newsroom, 2012.

16. Ibid.

17. Schröder, F.H., J. Hugosson, M.J. Roobol, T.L. Tammela, S. Ciatto, V. Nelen, M. Kwiatkowski, M. Lujan, H. Lilja, and M. Zappa, Screening and prostate-cancer mortality in a randomized European study. *New England Journal of Medicine*, 2009. **360**(13): p. 1320-1328.

18. Andriole, G. L., Crawford, E. D., Grubb III, R. L., Buys, S. S., Chia, D., Church, T. R., ... & Berg, C. D. Mortality Results From a Randomized Prostate Cancer Screening Trial. *New England Journal of Medicine*, **360**(13): p. 1310-19.

19. Bill-Axelson, A., L. Holmberg, M. Ruutu, M. Häggman, S.-O. Andersson, S. Bratell, A. Spångberg, C. Busch, S. Nordling, and H. Garmo, Radical prostatectomy versus watchful waiting in early prostate cancer. *New England Journal of Medicine*, 2005. **352**(19): p. 1977-1984.

20. Albertsen, P.C., J.A. Hanley, and J. Fine, 20-year outcomes following conservative management of clinically localized prostate cancer. *Journal American medical Association,* 2005. **293**(17): p. 2095-2101.

21. Johansson, J.-E., O. Andrén, S.-O. Andersson, P.W. Dickman, L. Holmberg, A. Magnuson, and H.-O. Adami, Natural history of early, localized prostate cancer. *JAMA,* 2004. **291**(22): p. 2713-2719.

22. Wilt, T.J., M.K. Brawer, K.M. Jones, M.J. Barry, W.J. Aronson, S. Fox, J.R. Gingrich, J.T. Wei, P. Gilhooly, and B.M. Grob, Radical prostatectomy versus observation for localized prostate cancer. *New England Journal of Medicine,* 2012. **367**(3): p. 203-213.

23. Wilt, T. J., and Brawer, M. K. The Prostate Cancer Intervention Versus Observation Trial: a randomized trial comparing radical prostatectomy versus expectant management for the treatment of clinically localized prostate cancer. *The Journal of uUrology,* 1994. **152**(5 Pt 2): 1910-1914.

24. Hamdy, F. *The protecT trial - evaluating the effectiveness of treatment for clinically localised prostate cancer.* 2013 [cited 2013 8/8/13]; Available from: http://www.hta.ac.uk/1230.

CHAPTER 6

Controversies in Mammography Screening

THE UNITED STATES Preventative Services Task Force, hereafter referred to as USPSTF, is a 10-member panel of nationally and internationally known experts in the various primary care specialties of internal and family medicine, pediatrics, obstetrics, and gynecology, as well as epidemiology. Although independent, the members are appointed by the federal government, specifically, the Department of Health and Human Services. Each member is appointed to a 4-year term with the possibility of an extension for an additional 1 to 2 years. The purpose of the Task Force is to review the latest available information concerning preventative services such as screening, vaccinations, *etc.* and to publish their recommendations periodically with on-going updates. The panel was first convened in 1984, completed its first set of recommendations in 1989, and has been providing updates since then.

Most recently, the USPSTF came under a considerable amount of criticism after it released its latest recommendations regarding mammography screening in November of 2009. In an apparent reversal of its 2002 recommendations that average-risk women, those without previous personal or first-degree family history (mother or sister) of breast cancer, receive screening starting at age 40 and repeat it every 1 to 2 years. The USPSTF recommended that screening begin at age 50 and, if normal, continue every two years. These new recommendations were based on new information; randomized clinical trials suggested that there was no evidence that screening women younger than 50 actually saved lives. I will return to this controversy in a bit more detail, but first a few words about the disease.

With the exception of skin cancer, breast cancer is the most commonly diagnosed malignancy in women. It is second only to lung cancer as a cause of cancer deaths. In 2010, an estimated 209,060 new cases were diagnosed and 40,330 deaths occurred (1). The risk of breast cancer increases with age, being relatively infrequent in women in their 30s and far more common in women between the ages of 45–65. This is the reason for being able to achieve a consensus for screening older women. The reason for screening is early detection, providing effective treatment and thereby preventing, or at least delaying, death. In previous chapters, we discussed a screening test's sensitivity — ability to identify those who truly have the disease — and its specificity — ability to identify those who do not have the disease. The sensitivity of mammography is 77–95%, whereas specificity is 94–97% (2). This variable sensitivity accounts for the many "false positives" that require women to return for repeat x-rays, sonograms, a newer technology known as digital mammography, and ultimately biopsy which, to date, is the only way to definitively diagnose cancer, by obtaining a piece of tissue and examining it under the microscope. False positives are actually quite common, particularly in younger women and overall, approximately one-third of mammograms in women between the ages of 40–49 result in false positives (3). This leads to anxiety, stress, radiation exposure, and ultimately the cost and discomfort of biopsy. With regard to radiation exposure — which is of particular concern to many women, the fear being that breast cancer can actually be caused by x-rays — that is a matter of some warranted concern.

To better understand how mammography could possibly be harmful, a few words about genetics would be helpful ... really. DNA is probably the most important molecule within the body because it provides the information that essentially instructs each cell in how to build tissues and organs. It carries information which determines our gender, eye color, and how many limbs we have. Radiation can increase the chance of disruption of the DNA molecule so that it can no longer do what it is supposed to do. A very high dose of radiation — 10, 000 rads, a unit of absorbed radiation — can cause death within 24–48 hours (4). The effect of radiation may not be to kill the cell, but rather to alter its genetic code in a way that leaves the cell alive but with an error in its blueprint (5). Cancer can therefore be produced if the error in the blueprint contributes to the loss of an important checkpoint thus causing the cell to divide uncontrollably and become a cancer (6). Theoretically, the more radiation exposure, the greater the potential for harm. "It is generally believed that there is no threshold below which cancerous rates would not be increased (7)." In other words, there is no definitive safe dose. Here, again, uncertainty raises its ugly head.

So we have established that breast cancer represents a significant public health problem. Because it tends to be slower-growing in older women (greater than 50 years old), it has a generally good prognosis. The 5-year survival rate; i.e. how many women are alive 5 years after diagnosis, is greater than 90% in cases of localized disease (8). Therefore, considering the criteria that we established in an earlier chapter to justify disease screening, breast cancer would appear appropriate for screening and few would disagree. So what is the basis for all of the controversy?

It is precisely because the development of breast cancer is age-related; the occurrence tends to rise precipitously after the age of 50 (9). General agreement exists in the orthodox medical community that screening women who are 50 or older is useful and evidence from trials indicates that lives are saved as a result (10). However, in 2009, the USPSTF recommended against routine screening of women aged 40–49, and that all women between 50–74 be screened every 2 years, instead of annually as previously recommended. Further, they advised against women examining their own breasts and they stated that the evidence was insufficient to argue for or against a clinical breast exam done by a medical professional. The new recommendations were motivated by the evidence of perceived harm from screening that more likely affected younger women. It was previously mentioned that the percentage of false positives was considerable, up to one-third of women between the ages 40–49. Based upon the criteria that we established in an earlier chapter, it would appear that mammography is indeed a good screening test, at least for older women. Breast cancer is a significant public health problem, accounting for approximately 40,000 deaths per year. An asymptomatic phase occurs first, when abnormalities can be detected by the test long before the patient is likely to have any complaints and, theoretically, treatments are available. The prognosis for a cure when the disease is early and localized is excellent (11). The test is relatively inexpensive (at least compared to colonoscopy) and, while many women complain of discomfort during the test (due to compression of the breasts), few would avoid repeating the test because of the discomfort. No one debates the advisability of women having what is referred to as a diagnostic mammogram, if she has symptoms suggestive of cancer such as a lump, pain or nipple discharge. Also, there are few who would argue against performing the test in a person with a close family history of breast cancer, genetic tests indicating high risk (so-called BRCA testing) or a personal history of DCIS (where a tumor was found in the milk ducts and is "in place," without the capacity to spread). Within the professional medical community little debate exists regarding the wisdom of screening in older women — 50 and above. The debate is whether lives are saved by conducting universal screening on asymptomatic women without high risk, who are younger than 50 years of age.

Although admittedly imperfect, the randomized clinical trial is probably the single most reliable instrument to answer clinical questions about large groups of people and, here, the critical question is whether mammography saves lives in younger women, thus justifying the performance of a test that is not completely without risks or harm. According to the National Cancer Institute (12) there are 5 potential harmful results of screening mammography:

1. Unnecessary follow-up procedures from false positives in which a mammogram shows a suspicious image, but there is actually no breast cancer.
2. A false sense of security from a false negative, because of a negative mammogram, *i.e.* one that doesn't reveal an abnormality when in fact breast cancer is present, might lead a person to ignore any change or symptom they might otherwise notice in their breasts.
3. Radiation — the effects of repeated exposure to radiation (such as annual screening mammograms) can build up over a lifetime, although admittedly this is of unknown precisely quantifiable significance.
4. Anxiety associated with waiting for results
5. Overdiagnosis — finding and treating a cancer or pre-cancerous condition such as DCIS that may not have ever been life threatening. We have no way of predicting which women with DCIS may later develop invasive cancer, which unlike the latter has the potential to spread.

Therefore the best available way to attempt to answer the critical question of screening's ability to save lives, is to examine the difference in survival rates in large groups of women — roughly half of those who have undergone screening and half who have not. Since 1963, there have been 8 large, randomized trials involving approximately a total of 641,000 women. Only the first of these trials, HIP of New York in 1963 (13) was conducted in the U.S., the others were in Sweden, Canada or the United Kingdom. Very few non-white or women over the age of 70 were involved. So once again, the ability to extrapolate to all women is highly questionable. The trials that are regarded as the most reliable and cited by the experts who compose the USPSTF are the Malmo (Swedish) trial of 1976 involving 42,283 women ages 45–69 (14) and the Canadian trial completed in 1993, involving 89,835 women between 40–59 years of age (15). In both trials, the women who received mammography screening had the same breast cancer death rate as the women who did not. The so-called Age Trial conducted in the United Kingdom in 2006 found a reduction in breast cancer death rate from screening during the 40s, but the finding was considered weak (16). In the language of statistics, the results were said to be *not* "statistically significant". In other words, the differences found could have been due to chance and not because of the intervention (screening).

In 2007, the American College of Physicians, an organization of 133,000 physicians, that represents the interests of 661, 400 physicians in the U.S. (2010 numbers), reviewed screening mammography studies in women 40–49 years of age. It included information from the original screening trials in addition to 117 other studies. They found rates of false-positive results as high as 20–56% after 10 years of mammograms, leading to increases in unnecessary procedures (17). The ACP reviewers, therefore, concluded that in the age group of 40–49, the risks of screening outweighed the advantages. In 1997, the National Cancer Institute concluded that the evidence was insufficient that screening women under 50 years of age would prevent cancer deaths (18). It should be pointed out that The American Cancer Society continues to recommend yearly mammograms starting at age 40 and continuing for as long as a woman is in "good health"(19).

With such variability in recommendations from different prestigious medical organizations very often looking at the same information, it is not surprising that there is confusion on the part of the general public and often among health professionals. In its 2002 recommendations, the USPSTF advised annual mammograms starting at age 40. The mission of the panel is to provide periodic updates based upon new information, however, patients become accustomed to previous patterns of behavior. If a woman has ever personally known or heard of someone diagnosed with breast cancer younger than age 50, it would be a much tougher sell to convince her to wait until she is 50. Laypersons have no knowledge of and often little interest in what "the literature" says. Furthermore, it is apparent that often professionals, who, presumably, do read the literature, are very much at odds. The recommendation against the practice of breast self-examinations was especially difficult to accept. Several primary care physicians, like myself, had spent the last 20 years advising and teaching patients how to examine their breasts and now we are told, "forget about it, it's a waste of time." Once again, randomized trials speak to and of large populations, not the individual sitting before you. What was found to be the case in Scandinavia or England (or even in someone down the street) may have nothing to do with you. When the updated recommendations were announced, several women questioned the motivation behind them. Was the USPSTF in collusion with the insurance industry? Are they just trying to save the industry money, because they just don't want to pay for the mammograms? Given the general culpability and justifiably poor credibility of the insurance industry, this is not an unreasonable conclusion. It is more plausible, however, that the relatively "independent" practitioners and researchers on the panel were more likely influenced by their reading of the data from the trials. Also, the recommendations are felt to be the most reasonable for the *general* population. The Task Force recognizes that each practitioner will advocate for what makes sense in their individual patient population.

It must be repeated, in every chapter if necessary, that medicine is a people business. It is flawed and imperfect. Evidence is not absolute and is subject to various interpretations in light of individual and varied experiences. Based upon my 3 decades in clinical medicine, my approach is, and has always been that recommendations are to be given on an individual basis. Whether it be mammography or any other form of screening, patients should be made aware of the pros and cons of any potential intervention. They should be informed of the little of which is "known", the much of which is "believed," the reality that generalizations can be risky, at best, and that they need to get used to being prepared to accept the consequences of *their* choices, which need to be as informed as possible. Here, it is the responsibility of the health care professional to provide or at least introduce that information and explain it clearly to the extent that the patient cares to know.

References Cited

1. Jemal, A., R. Siegel, J. Xu, and E. Ward, Cancer statistics, *CA: A Cancer Journal for Clinicians*, 2010. **60**(5): p. 277-300.
2. Nelson, H.D., K. Tyne, A. Naik, C. Bougatsos, B.K. Chan, and L. Humphrey, Screening for breast cancer: an update for the US Preventive Services Task Force. *Annals of Internal Medicine*, 2009. **151**(10): p. 727-737.
3. *Breast Cancer Screening Health Professional Version*. 2013 [cited 2013 August 28, 2013]; Available from: http://www.cancer.gov/cancertopics/pdq/screening/breast/healthprofessional.
4. Faden, R.R., Final Report of the Advisory Committee on Human Radiation Experiments. Washington, DC: US Government Printing Office, 1995. p.3
5. Ibid.
6. Ibid.

7. Ibid.p.5.

8. *Breast Cancer Overview.* 2013 [cited 2013 April 24]; Available from: http://www.cancer.org/cancer/breastcancer/overviewguide/breast-cancer-overview-key-statistics.

9. *Risk Factors for Breast Cancer.* 2011 [cited 2013 June 23]; Available from: http://www.health.harvard.edu/newsletters/Harvard Womens Health Watch/2011/October/risk-factors-for-breast-cancer.

10. Nelson, H. D., Tyne, K., Naik, A., Bougatsos, C., Chan, B. K., and Humphrey, L. Screening for breast cancer: an update for the US Preventive Services Task Force. 2009. *Annals of Internal Medicine, 151*(10), 727-737.

11. Breast Cancer Overview. 2013 [cited 2013 July 9]; Available from: http://www.cancer.org/cancer/breastcancer/overviewguide/

12. NCI. *National Cancer Advisory Board Issues Mammography Screening Recommendations.* 1997 [cited 2013 August 1]; Available from: http://www.nih.gov/news/pr/mar97/nci-27b.htm.

13. Shapiro, S., W. Venet, P. Strax, L. Venet, and R. Roeser, Selection, follow-up, and analysis in the Health Insurance Plan Study: a randomized trial with breast cancer screening. *National Cancer Institute Monograph*, 1985. **67**: p. 65-74.

14. Andersson, I., K. Aspegren, L. Janzon, T. Landberg, K. Lindholm, F. Linell, O. Ljungberg, J. Ranstam, and B. Sigfusson, Mammographic screening and mortality from breast cancer: the Malmö mammographic screening trial. *British Medical Journal*, 1988. **297**(6654): p. 943.

15. Miller, A.B., T. To, C.J. Baines, and C. Wall, The Canadian National Breast Screening Study-1: breast cancer mortality after 11 to 16 years of follow-up: a randomized screening trial of mammography in women age 40 to 49 years. *Annals of Internal Medicine*, 2002. **137**(5_Part_1): p. 305-312.

16. Johns, L. and S. Moss, Randomized controlled trial of

mammographic screening from age 40 ('Age'trial): patterns of screening attendance. *Journal of Medical Screening*, 2010. **17**(1): p. 37-43.

17. *New Guideline for Screening Mammography for Women 40 to 49 Years of Age.* 2007 [cited 2013 Februrary 16]; Available from: http://www.acponline.org/pressroom/mam_guideline.htm.

18. National Cancer Advisory Board Issues Mammography Screening Recommendations. NIH News Release. March 27, 1997: Available from: http://www.nih.gov/news/pr/mar97/nci-27b.htm

19. *American Cancer Society recommendations for early breast cancer detection in women without breast symptoms.* 2013 [cited 2013 June 21]; Available from: http://www.cancer.org/cancer/breastcancer/moreinformation/breastcancerearlydetection/breast-cancer-early-detection-acs-recs.

CHAPTER 7

Immunization Practices

WITH RARE EXCEPTION every recommendation coming from the established medical community in this country is met with some opposition, especially if it is in the area of prevention. Less controversy is generated concerning the treatment of documented diseases. On the other hand, convincing people to submit to the injection of foreign material into their bodies with the hope of preventing a disease that is either not commonly seen today or perceived as being trivial, is difficult. This is even more difficult if there have been at least anecdotal reports of disabling or, at worst, lethal side effects. Few medical recommendations from the medical establishment have been met with as much impassioned opposition as that of universal vaccinations.

The panel that has the responsibility of making vaccine recommendations is the Advisory Committee on Immunization Practices (ACIP), the members of which are appointed by the Secretary of the Department of Health and Human Services. The panel consists of 15 regular members who are considered expert in one of several fields including clinical and laboratory vaccine research; safety and efficacy; use of vaccines in clinical practice or preventative medicine; and social and community aspects of immunization programs. In addition to the regular members there are 8 ex-officio members representing federal agencies that have the responsibility for administering immunization programs and 30 non-voting representatives of liaison organizations that have related immunization expertise. The panel meets three times per year and reviews the morbidity and mortality — illnesses and deaths — caused by diseases that are preventable by vaccination. They also study the scientific literature on safety and efficacy of vaccines, the recommendations of other groups, the labeling and package inserts of vaccine manufactures and the feasibility of vaccine use in existing programs. The mission of the ACIP is to provide advice to government agencies for reducing the incidence of vaccine-preventable diseases. The ACIP statements represent the official federal recommendations and are published by the CDC.

One might wonder why there is such distrust of the recommendations provided by such a seemingly august body as the ACIP. A few words of explanation are in order at this point. Probably the principal reason why so much distrust of government and medical establishment recommendations exists is because of the role of money in virtually every aspect of our daily lives. The corrupting influence that money has in our politics can be appreciated by most of us. The fact that the medical industry, which, in my view, is controlled to a great extent by the private insurance industry and is driven by the profit motive is certainly apparent to those of us who have spent several years in the field, if not in the academy or the laboratory. The full implementation of The Affordable Care Act (Obamacare) in 2014 has not diminished the power of the industry as it receives millions of previously uninsured customers. The fact that some clinicians and scientists can, in fact, be purchased — the polite term is they have apparent conflicts of interests — helps to erode confidence and makes the less gullible among us suspicious when we hear that it is recommended that virtually *everyone* receive a given intervention, in this case, vaccinations.

Vaccines are injections or oral administrations of either a killed or weakened form of the germ purported to cause the disease that the vaccine is meant to protect against. Through an intricate and magnificent network known as our immune system, the vaccines are said to work by causing specialized cells to develop antibodies, which are proteins that protect the body from disease if it is exposed. In the interest of brevity suffice it to say that the purpose of the immune system is to recognize *self* from *non-self* — tumors, viruses, bacteria, *etc.* that do not naturally belong in *self.* The vaccine contains substances that mimic the actual — natural — infection so that if exposed to the germ that causes, for example, flu, hepatitis, or measles, the immune system's "memory cells " will recognize this foreign invader — non-self — and attack and eliminate it. Of course, if the immune system is weakened due to inadequate nutrition or exercise; excessive alcohol or other drugs, legal or illegal; then this intricate network of cells may not work as well and one is more likely to become ill if exposed to the disease-causing germ in question.

The concept of vaccination, or inoculation, was known at least as long ago as 17th century China, as noted in a 1913 text by the International Congress of Medicine (1); however, in recent times, the one who is often credited with development of the modern vaccine, particularly against smallpox, was a British country doctor named Edward Jenner. Jenner noted that young women who milked cows developed a rash on their hands, similar to smallpox in appearance, known as cowpox, and that, curiously, these women never developed smallpox, which was epidemic in that British community at the time. Jenner extracted the liquid from a young woman's sores and also the liquid from the sores of another person who had a mild form of smallpox. He felt that if he could inject someone with cowpox, the germs from the relatively mild cowpox would enable the person's body to defend itself against the dangerous smallpox germs, which he planned to inject later. Reportedly, Jenner convinced a farmer to allow him to inject his young son, which incredibly he agreed to (talk about being a guinea pig). Jenner made an incision on the child's arm and injected the cowpox material and covered the arm. The child developed mild symptoms of cowpox. Jenner later injected the child with smallpox and noted that he never became ill. This was an extremely dangerous experiment that could have resulted in his being charged with murder had the child died as most did during that period. Instead, he is regarded as a pioneer of a technique that ultimately is credited with greatly contributing to the worldwide eradication of smallpox, which was declared by the World Health Organization in 1979, when the last case was reported.

> Smallpox is a contagious disease, unique to humans, caused by a virus and characterized by a pustular rash with long-term complications such as severe scaring, limb deformities and blindness in as much as one-third of its victims. In the past, the death rate from the disease was anywhere from 20 to 60% and as much as 80% in children (24). The disease was known to humans as far back as 10 thousand years prior to the Christian era (25). It was reportedly first identified, or at least its characteristic rash, in the mummified remains of the Egyptian Pharaoh, Ramses V over 3000 years ago (26). The disease killed an estimated 400 thousand Europeans in the 18th century (27).

Jenner conducted his first "human experiments" in 1796 and published his results 2 years later, however, there was very little in the way of vaccine development for almost the next one hundred years. French Biologist, Louis Pasteur proposed the Germ Theory in 1877, which today is regarded as a well-established principle of medicine and is a cornerstone of public health sanitation policy. All of those among us who have prescribed and/or taken antibiotics certainly accept this theory. Virtually all concepts in medicine have been the subject of challenge and controversy — including the Germ Theory. It is beyond the scope of this chapter to discuss every controversy and its basis. Suffice it to say that not everyone buys this theory, which basically states that infectious diseases are caused by microscopic organisms such as bacteria, viruses and fungi. In his day, Pasteur's claims were challenged by another French biologist, Antoine Béchamp who maintained that microorganisms, specifically bacteria, were capable of changing form and did not, in fact, cause but were produced *by* disease, arising from tissues that had been damaged by enzymes— substances that are produced by all living organisms that speed up chemical processes, such as digestion, in the body. An older contemporary of Pasteur and Béchamp, French Physiologist, Claude Bernard maintained that what was critical was not the germ, but the terrain, as he termed it, the "internal milieu." Today we might say that what is most important is not the disease-causing agent, the microorganism, but rather the host, the one who is being infected. On some level, most of us can relate to this concept because we recognize that everyone is not equally affected by a reputed disease-causing organism. It is the strength of our immune system that may determine our response to the invading organism and even our outcome. This is relevant in light of the objections of many who oppose mandatory vaccinations, contending that if we maintain good health we can withstand any potential for illness from organisms to which we become exposed.

In 1900, only one vaccine — smallpox — was given to children. By the 1950s, it was up to four. Since the 1980s several have been added and as of June of 2011, 27 vaccine-preventable diseases have been acknowledged by the WHO and the CDC. The CDC recommends vaccination against 16 diseases in 12 injections be given routinely (2).

During this greater than 200-year history, the grounds for objection to vaccination remained consistent. Critics have maintained that vaccines represent foreign and poisonous material that can cause adverse reactions worse than the diseases they are attempting to prevent;

that they simply don't work; that forcing individuals to take them represents a violation of individual liberties and religious or philosophical beliefs. Further, some claim that improving personal hygiene and good nutrition can give a more natural and lasting immunity.

The rationale for vaccination, or inoculation, as the terms are sometimes used interchangeably, was advanced several decades before Jenner's experiments. In 1721, Reverend Cotton Mather introduced inoculation to Boston, Massachusetts during a smallpox epidemic. Although there were considerable religious objections, he was able to convince a Dr. Boylston to experiment with the approach. The approach consisted of making small incisions in the arm of a person, applying fluid from the sores of small pox sufferers and covering the area. Boylston experimented on his six year old son; his slave; and the son of the slave. Each person developed the disease, became ill for a period but, as he later wrote, "after several days, the sickness vanished and they were no longer gravely ill." (3). Religious objections were given at the time. In a 1722 sermon entitled "The Dangerous and Sinful Practice of Inoculation," the English theologian, Reverend Edmund Massey stated that diseases were sent by God to punish sin and that any attempt to prevent smallpox by way of inoculation was a "diabolic operation" (4).

For many opponents of vaccination, the marked diminution or eradication of various infectious diseases could be attributed to several factors other than the vaccine:

1. Many of the vaccine-preventable diseases were said actually to have been in decline prior to the introduction of the vaccine (5).
2. Improvements in sanitation, hygiene and water quality and adequate food (6).
3. Increase in access to birth control methods (7).
4. Reduction in poverty and overcrowding (8).

It is difficult to say with certainty that an intervention designed to prevent a disease has actually been effective, in any given individual. If the individual does not, in fact, develop the condition after using the measure, we can only get a suggestion of efficacy by looking at communities.

Between 1873–74 in Stockholm, Sweden, an anti-vaccination campaign motivated by religious concerns, questions about vaccine efficacy and the rights of individuals, led to the vaccination rate dropping to 40% compared to about 90% in other parts of Sweden. A major smallpox epidemic then developed in 1873 that triggered an increase in vaccine use and the subsequent end of the epidemic (9).

In 1974, a report in the United Kingdom attributed severe adverse reactions to the pertussis (whooping cough) vaccine. Prominent public health officials openly questioned the efficacy and suggested that more harm than benefit resulted from its use. Vaccine use dropped from 81% to 31% and an epidemic ensued, resulting in some children's deaths. After a national reassessment of vaccine safety and efficacy, the public confidence was ultimately restored. Vaccine rates again rose to greater than 90% and disease incidence dropped dramatically (10).

When Sweden suspended its vaccination program against pertussis from 1979–1996, 60% of the country's children developed this potentially fatal disease. In many parts of the world where mass vaccination is not practiced, pertussis continues to be a major health problem. According to the WHO, the disease was responsible for 294,000 deaths in 2002 (11).

The measles outbreak in The Netherlands from 1999–2000 illustrates that even relatively developed countries may not be spared from communicable disease epidemics. The population in several of the affected communities had high rates of immunization except for one religious denomination who traditionally did not accept vaccination. Three measles-related deaths and 68 hospitalizations occurred in that particular unvaccinated community (12).

In 1998, the British medical publication, *The Lancet*, published an article by a physician, Andrew Wakefield, which attributed the development of autism in 12 children to the measles, mumps, rubella (MMR) vaccine, primarily based upon the observation that the children developed the symptoms soon after having received the vaccine. Wakefield suggested that giving 3 vaccines individually would be safer than providing one "umbrella" injection, although he failed to provide evidence for this. It was later learned that Wakefield received funding from lawyers who were representing parents involved in litigation against the vaccine manufacturers. The author apparently failed to disclose this conflict of interest. The article was ultimately determined to be fraudulent, 11 of the co-authors withdrew their names from the publication and *The Lancet* published a retraction in 2010. Wakefield lost his license to practice medicine in Great Britain. As a result of the MMR controversy, the vaccination rates dropped dramatically, below 80% throughout the commonwealth and as low as 60% in parts of North Dublin. There were 300 reported cases of measles with 100 hospitalization and three deaths. Some of those hospitalized required mechanical ventilation (13).

In the first few years of this century, some religious leaders in northern Nigeria, suspicious of Western medicine, advised their followers not to have their children vaccinated with the polio vaccine. With the support of the governor of the state of Kano, immunization was suspended for several months. Subsequently, polio reappeared in several formerly polio-free communities in Nigeria and genetic testing demonstrated that the virus was one that originated in northern Nigeria. Nigeria had now become an exporter of polio to some of its neighbors on the continent. People in the northern states were also suspicious of other vaccines and from January through March of 2005, Nigeria reported over 20,000 cases of measles with close to 600 deaths. In 2006, Nigeria accounted for over half of the new cases of polio worldwide (14). Outbreaks continued unabated; in 2007 at least 200 children died in a measles outbreak in the Nigerian state of Borno (15).

In the United States in 2005, the CDC attributed an outbreak of measles in the state of Indiana to children that went unvaccinated because their parents had refused to allow it (16). Tetanus is a disease that few of us in this country have any experience with, however, most cases of pediatric tetanus in the U.S. occur in children whose parents objected to their vaccination.

So, do the above examples "prove" the efficacy of vaccines and could continued opposition to public health programs spell disaster? The evidence, albeit imperfect, suggests that the answer is yes. Medicine and epidemiology are not exact sciences and "proof" is a term used too often. Data only suggest reality, some data suggest more convincingly than others. In terms of vaccine efficacy, we can only compare vaccinated with unvaccinated populations with respect to the disease in question. In terms of safety, the history of vaccinations would certainly give cause for concern if we consider how the vaccines were prepared in the pre-germ theory era. The risks of skin infections from such treatments were real.

Distrust of government is not totally without merit. The legacy of the Tuskegee syphilis study (17) comes to mind, as do the CIA experiments with LSD on American soldiers (18). However, at the risk of appearing naïve, I would like to think that we live in somewhat less barbaric times and that the evidence is certainly insufficient to suggest that the government would on a grand scale deliberately poison its own citizens, not to mention encourage the poisoning be carried out worldwide. The CDC has erred in the past (19) but they are not the enemy at this time. The quality control that is utilized to ensure the safety of vaccines is impressive. Admittedly, the reporting of adverse reactions to vaccines is flawed very probably because most doctors are convinced of the safety of the agents — although there is evidence that younger physicians tend to be more skeptical (20). Therefore, if a child or adult develops an illness in close proximity to having received an injection, many doctors would very likely declare that the two events were unrelated and the illness likely would not be reported as an adverse effect. Much of the distrust of vaccines in recent times comes from older people who remember the swine flu scare and the vaccine, which, at that time was associated with several illnesses. There were reportedly 500 cases of Guillain-Barre syndrome, a potentially paralyzing disease, in 1976, and at least three deaths of elderly people who received the injection. Was the injection the cause or were they three elderly people who, not surprisingly, died of heart disease, the leading cause of death in the elderly?

During my nearly 30 years in private medical practice, I have spoken with scores of patients who swore they would never take the flu shot because they had the shot "in the 1970s and got sick as a dog." Did they really? I certainly don't know. Could it be that the vaccine was ineffective and they just got the flu and assumed that the vaccine made them ill?

Populations appear to benefit from vaccination. There appears to be some validity to the concept of herd immunity. This type of protection is presumed to be given to unvaccinated individuals in a community if a significant percentage of that community has been vaccinated. A recent example of this concept was illustrated in a Canadian study published in the *Journal of the AMA* (21). However, in a given individual, it is not at all clear how protective, for example, the flu vaccine is. There is anecdotal information from my own practice, and yes it is only anecdotal, but that too has power of a sort; I've had many patients who never get vaccinated, never get the flu, others who get vaccinated and still get the flu. Of course, supporters of mass vaccination would probably say that, well, yes they still got the flu but they didn't get as ill as they would have if they had not been vaccinated — pure speculation. We have no idea of what would have happened to that *individual* if they were not vaccinated. So what am I suggesting? Generally, I am very much pro-vaccination. I believe that the evidence, worldwide, is that vaccinations can save lives and minimize serious illness; however, as with so many things, especially in this country, entirely too much hype and scare tactics are used to force people into line. The 1976 swine flu scare is an example, where a threatened plague never materialized and perhaps more suffered from the vaccine than the actual infection in that year. Also the 2009 swine flu scare was similarly overdone. The great flu of 1918, which killed 20–30 million people worldwide in less than a year (22) and further debilitated millions more, probably provides the rationale for such hysteria. The CDC and other public health officials are responsible for the "PUBLIC" so, understandably, they have to take a broad stroke approach and recommend measures that promise to protect large numbers of people. Practically, there would be major political fall-out if they failed to be aggressive and large numbers of the population were jeopardized. So they can't afford to get it wrong. President Gerald Ford's determination to vaccinate the entire population against a plague that never materialized and possibly resulted in the disability of hundreds may have played a role in his failure to win re-election. For those who say that these issues are above politics, there is no such thing!

Even though the concept of herd immunity has validity, individuals must still be given the opportunity to refuse vaccination, for religious or philosophical reasons. Their rationale may sometimes be shown to be patently irrational, but again, on an individual level, specific outcomes are not always predictable and people must certainly retain the right to be foolish and accept responsibility for their choices. Also skepticism of perceived wisdom, be it from government, academics, or industries, is healthy and grounded in reality, as indicated by a few of the examples above. The reality is we do not know what causes autism, and if you are the parent of a child who develops signs and symptoms of autism soon after receiving a vaccination, all of the scientific studies in the world will not be sufficient to dissuade you from the belief that there was a causal connection. The medical establishment, therefore, needs to be more understanding and less dismissive. It may very well be that the vaccine or an infection — viral or otherwise — may, in an individual who is genetically predisposed, be the trigger that allows the condition to express itself. The point is, as is often the case, we don't know. The role of the anti-vaccinationists may appear disruptive, wrongheaded, and often patently irresponsible, particularly with respect to their position on childhood vaccines. It is wise, however, to at least question the proliferation of yet more vaccines and not merely submit to the scare tactics used by the media and sponsored by the government and vaccine manufacturers. If the arguments of the anti-vaccinationists are flawed, they need to be challenged with at least epidemiological evidence as noted in the discussion of the worldwide measles outbreak. Another example of a responsible rebuff to the contrarians was offered by the 2002 Institute of Medicine Immunization Safety review that refuted the notion that infants received more vaccines than was necessary (23). However, no review of any number of studies will ever quiet the concerns of everyone, but the challenge should more closely resemble the often-touted evidence-based approach rather than mere ridicule and dismissal.

References Cited

1. Burroughs Wellcome and Company. [from old catalog], The history of inoculation and vaccination for the prevention and treatment of disease; lecture memoranda, American Medical Association, 1913. 1913, London: Burroughs Wellcome & Co.
2. Bridges, C.B., M.L. Woods, and T. Coyne-Beasley, Advisory Committee on Immunization Practices (ACIP) Recommended Immunization Schedule for Adults Aged 19 Years and Older—United States, 2013. Morbidity and mortality weekly report. Surveillance summaries (Washington, DC: 2002), 2013. 62(1): p. 9-19.

3. Allen, A., *Vaccine: The Controversial Story of Medicine's Greatest Lifesaver*. 2007, New York: W.W. Norton & Company.

4. White, A.D., Theological Opposition to Inoculation, Vaccination and the Use of Anesthetics, in *A History of the Warfare of Science with Theology in Christendom*. 1896, D. Appleton and Company: New York.

5. Null, G. *Vaccines: A Second Opinion*. pp.14-16

6. Ibid.

7. Starr, P., *The Social Transformation of American Medicine*. 1982, New York: Basic Books. p.135.

8. *The Vaccination Inquirer and Health Review*. 1880, London: Edward D. Allen.p.157.

9. Nelson, M. C., and Rogers, J. (1992). The right to die? Anti-vaccination activity and the 1874 smallpox epidemic in Stockholm. *Social History of Medicine*, 5(3), 369-388.

10. Gangarosa, E.J., A. Galazka, C. Wolfe, L. Phillips, R. Gangarosa, E. Miller, and R. Chen, Impact of anti-vaccine movements on pertussis control: the untold story. *The Lancet*, 1998. 351(9099): p. 356-361.

11. Epidemiology and Prevention of Vaccine-Preventable Diseases. *The Pink Book: Course Textbook, in Epidemiology and Prevention of Vaccine-Preventable Diseases* The 2012, Centers for Disease Control and Prevention: Atlanta, GA.

12. van den Hof, S., C. Meffre, M. Conyn-van Spaendonck, F. Woonink, H.E. de Melker, and R.S. van Binnendijk, Measles outbreak in a community with very low vaccine coverage, the Netherlands. *Emerging Infectious Diseases*, 2001. 7(3 Suppl): p. 593.

13. Pepys, M.B., Science and serendipity. *Clinical Medicine*, 2007. 7(6): p. 562-578.

14. NIGERIA: Children dying needlessly from measles and other preventable diseases. IRIN, the humanitatrian news and analysis

service of the UN Office for the cooridination of Humanitarian Affairs., 2007.

15. Michael, O., Nigeria: Measles Outbreak-Borno's Harvest of Death. This Day (Lagos) OPINION, 2007. 21.

16. Import-Associated Measles Outbreak --- Indiana, May--June 2005. MMWR 2005; Available from: http://www.cdc.gov/mmwr/preview/mmwrhtml/mm5442a1.htm.

17. Jones, J.H., *Bad Blood: the Tuskegee Syphilis Experiment.* New York: Free Press, 2003.

18. Price, D.H., Buying a piece of anthropology. *Anthropology Today,* 2007. 23(5): p. 17-22.

19. Historical Perspectives History of CDC. *Morbidity and Mortality Weekly Report,* 1996. 45(25): p. 526-530.

20. Laino, C. Survey: Younger Doctors More Skeptical of Vaccines. 2011 [cited 2013 July 11]; Available from: http://children.webmd.com/vaccines/news/20111021/survey-younger-doctors-more-skeptical-of-vaccines.

21. Loeb, M., M.L. Russell, L. Moss, K. Fonseca, J. Fox, D.J. Earn, F. Aoki, G. Horsman, P. Van Caeseele, and K. Chokani, Effect of influenza vaccination of children on infection rates in Hutterite communities. *Journal of the American Medical Association,* 2010. 303(10): p. 943-950.

22. Billings, M., The influenza pandemic of 1918. 1997 [cited 2013 July 14]; Available from: http://virus.stanford.edu/uda/.

23. Stratton, K.R., C.B. Wilson, and M.C. McKormick, Immunization Safety Review: Multiple Immunizations and Immune Dysfunction. Washington D.C.: National Academies Press, 2002.

24. Riedel, S., Edward Jenner and the history of smallpox and vaccination. *Proceedings Baylor University. Medical Center,* 2005. 18(1): p. 21.

25. Ibid.

26. Ibid.

27. Ibid.

CHAPTER 8

The Lipid Hypothesis

ANYONE WHO HAS been keeping up with the medical news, even in the popular press, is by now, aware of the huge impact that heart disease has on public health. Approximately 150,000 people develop heart attacks in the United States every year with one-third being fatal. Most of us are probably also aware of some of the risk factors — those conditions putting one at increased risk for heart disease — high blood pressure, cigarette smoking, diabetes, family history, possibly obesity, and high cholesterol. Most of us in the medical community, those who take care of patients on a daily basis and virtually all of the general public, accept this list of risk factors as legitimate. In over 30 years of medical practice, I don't recall anyone, in print or elsewhere, touting the virtues of hypertension, diabetes or cigarettes. The importance of cholesterol, however, remains a subject of debate. The lipid hypothesis does not maintain that high cholesterol is the only causative factor in the development of heart disease. In the words of Dr. Daniel Steinberg, "the lipid hypothesis does propose that hypercholesterolemia is the determining factor, *i.e.* it is sufficiently dominant that correcting it will significantly reduce the burden of disease and its clinical consequences even if the cholesterol is the sole variable manipulated"(1). If you read most of the literature readily available in this country, professional or lay; listen to the masses of medical "experts," be they orthodox or alternative/complementary; or watch the various TV commercials for one or another cholesterol-lowering drug, one would presume that the lipid or cholesterol hypothesis is a slam dunk. At this time, I should explain briefly what this hypothesis is and what evidence has been presented over the years to support or refute it.

Atherosclerosis (arteriosclerosis) is a chronic disease characterized by a hardening of the arteries, beginning early in life, progressing with age, and thought, by most, to be contributed to by lipid or fat found in the blood. Over time, the arteries are presumed to be clogged by this fat, reducing the flow of blood to the heart, brain, legs, and wherever else blood is carried throughout the body. The classic teaching, and what I have always told my patients, is that blood carries oxygen and nutrients, and if the flow of blood is impeded, a condition known as ischemia can develop in the area deprived of these nutrients which can ultimately result in infarction, or tissue death. If this occurs in the heart, a heart attack ensues, in the brain, a stroke. If the process occurs in the arteries going to the kidneys, failure can develop, requiring dialysis or transplant and if in the legs it can lead to discoloration, pain and disability. Virtually everyone in the scientific community agrees on the definition and consequences of atherosclerosis, but not everyone accepts the role of dietary fat. The proponents of the lipid hypothesis further maintain that if the cholesterol level measured in the blood is high — the acceptable levels to be determined periodically by "expert panels" — then you are at greater risk for atherosclerosis and its consequences. The hypothesis further implies that lowering the cholesterol level reduces risk.

During the past 20 years, greater emphasis has been placed on the distinction between the so-called "good" and "bad" cholesterol. In the interest of simplicity, the HDL is considered good because it carries lipids (fats) away from the heart where it is ultimately transported to the gastrointestinal system and eliminated from the body. The LDL is said to be bad because it carries lipids back to the heart. The level of good cholesterol does not change that dramatically with diet or drugs, but can be increased minimally with exercise. The bad component can be decreased somewhat with diet, but most dramatically with medications, especially the newer class of agents known as statins.

The statins (Mevacor®, Lipitor®, and Crestor®, for example), the newest and most effective class of drugs available for lowering the cholesterol level, work by interfering with a critical step in the production of cholesterol. The first statin was discovered by Akira Endo in 1976 in the laboratory of the Sanyko pharmaceutical company in Tokyo.

The proponents of the lipid hypothesis are confident of the truth of their conclusions primarily because of what they feel to be the "totality of the evidence" (2). The various lines or categories of evidence include 1) experimental or animal data; 2) genetic analysis; 3) findings from epidemiological studies; and 4) the results of clinical trials. One of the strongest arguments in favor of the hypothesis is offered in the 2007 publication of *The Cholesterol Wars: The Skeptics Vs. the Preponderance of Evidence* by Daniel Steinberg. He has especially compelling establishment credentials as Professor of Medicine Emeritus at the University of California, San Diego; he has also authored some 400 scientific articles on lipids and atherosclerosis; and he served in a leadership capacity on the 1984 Lipids Research Panel that promulgated the modern recommendations regarding the monitoring and treatment of hypercholesterolemia. It is because of Steinberg's prominent role as a "thought leader" in the field that I will use most of the evidence offered in his book in support of the hypothesis to exemplify the proponents' position on this controversy.

Russian pathologist, Nikolai Anitschkow (1885–1964) is credited with providing the most thorough and convincing data on the role of cholesterol in the development of atherosclerosis. In 1913, he and his associates demonstrated that feeding rabbits cholesterol (in the form of egg yolks) produced damage to blood vessels closely resembling that of human atherosclerosis. They were able to duplicate their experiments and also noted that the extent of the damage was directly correlated to the level of cholesterol elevation in the blood of the experimental animals. Furthermore, when the egg yolk diet was stopped after a few months and the animals' usual plant-based diet was resumed, the damage was reversed. Steinberg points out that many other investigators at the time did not accept Anitschkow's findings because they were unable to duplicate the experiment in their laboratories with rats or dogs. Steinberg points out that what was not appreciated in the early years of Anitschkow's experiments was that rats and dogs, unlike rabbits, have evolved a very efficient system for converting dietary cholesterol to bile acids, thereby being able to eliminate it through the stool. Therefore, despite being fed large amounts of high-fat foods, their blood cholesterol was, at best, minimally elevated. Anitschkow's experiments were carried on for approximately 50 years and over time he was able to demonstrate that atherosclerosis could be induced in several different animal species provided that the blood cholesterol levels could be sufficiently elevated and over a long enough period of time. Toward the end of Steinberg's chapter on animal models of experimental atherosclerosis, he provides a table listing over a dozen species, including dogs, cats, monkeys, and pigs in which atherosclerosis has been induced by increasing blood cholesterol levels (3).

DNA is the hereditary material in human beings and virtually all other organisms. The information in DNA is stored as a code made up of 4 chemicals that are most simply designated as A, G, C, and T. Their sequence order determines the information available for building and maintaining an individual, for example, hair, eye, and skin color. In a similar fashion, the letters in the alphabet are sequenced to form words or sentences. A mutation is a permanent change in the DNA sequence that makes up a gene. These mutations can either be inherited from a parent or acquired during a lifetime due to environmental factors such as radiation. Familial hypercholesterolemia (FH) is caused by a mutation of the LDL receptor. This receptor is an apparatus located on the surface of the cell. Its role is to draw cholesterol from the blood into the cell to make the vitamins and hormones needed by the body. If there isn't enough cholesterol taken into the cells, it builds up in the blood, and as it travels through the arteries, it ultimately clogs the tubing. As per the hypothesis, this leads to atherosclerosis and the complications we spoke of earlier. One of these often-associated complications can be the development of xanthomas.

Xanthomas are firm, often yellowish deposits that occur usually just under the skin of the legs or arms, and occasionally on the face. In *The Cholesterol Wars*, Steinberg noted that in 1889 Lehzen and Knauss reported the case of a child who had several xanthomas throughout her body since the age of 3 and who died suddenly at 11. The autopsy examination revealed extensive xanthoma deposits in the aorta and other large arteries, including the coronary arteries. Her 9-year-old sister also reportedly had xanthomas under the skin. The significance of these deposits was debated for several years thereafter but later scientists were able to demonstrate that the presence of these deposits was often accompanied by elevated cholesterol in the blood and that the xanthoma itself actually contained stored cholesterol. In retrospect, it is felt that the two sisters described above actually had familial hypercholesterolemia. The form of the condition that the sisters had is admittedly rare, occurring in approximately one in a million births; however, there is a more common variant said to occur in about one in 500 births. In 1939, Carl Mueller, a professor of internal medicine, based upon a study of 76 cases in 17 Norwegian families was reportedly the first to publish evidence that linked xanthomas of the skin to high cholesterol in the blood and coronary artery disease (4). It is now argued, and perhaps quite convincingly, that with the introduction of statin therapy many of these FH patients can be spared an early death as was experienced by the young girls mentioned earlier. It is certainly clear and without controversy that statins can markedly reduce cholesterol levels in the blood. These patients tend to have extraordinarily high values. I clearly remember taking care of two teen family members in the 1990s, who routinely had cholesterol values close to 500, which was reduced by 50 to 75% by medication.

The epidemiological evidence offered by the proponents of the hypothesis is probably the most controversial, though most often cited. As we defined it in an earlier chapter, epidemiology is the study of disease in populations; it specifically is concerned with how, when, and where disease occurs. Epidemiological studies can only provide evidence that a risk factor(s) is correlated with a disease, but not that it causes the disease.

A typical and often cited example of an epidemiological study is one that studies the effects of tobacco use. A researcher might recruit two groups of individuals — smokers and non-smokers — without evidence of cancer. They monitor these individuals over time and determine at the end of the study period if the groups differ in the prevalence of the outcome of interest, for example, lung or oral cancer. To make this more interesting, let's say that this study was conducted 40–50 years ago when the evidence for the carcinogenic effects of tobacco was less overwhelming than today. If the results of the study demonstrated that there was a greater prevalence of cancer in the group of smokers, a *correlation* between smoking and cancer would have been established, but not *proof of causation*. Virtually every week, the popular media reports a study that demonstrates some correlation between a behavior and a disease. Just recently, I heard of a report revealing a correlation between hair relaxers and uterine fibroids (5). Epidemiological studies, showing correlations may *suggest* causation, but no more. This type of study is said to be *observational*. The problem with such a study is that the groups being observed usually differ in ways in addition to the risk factor that is being studied. Using the example above, smokers and non-smokers may have differing characteristics or behaviors other than tobacco exposure that can affect their likelihood of developing cancer, such as family history, alcohol intake, diet, level of physical activity, gender, or ethnicity. These other factors that may impact the outcome are referred to as "confounders". Sophisticated statistical analysis can be used to remove the effect of known confounders. Unknown or un-measured confounders, where the investigators are unable to control for or take into account can unknowingly affect the study. Despite the flaws of this study type we have gained invaluable information over the years concerning human disease. The following are some examples of observational evidence that is often offered by the proponents of the cholesterol hypothesis.

In the 1950s, Ancel Keys, a scientist from the University of Minnesota, was reportedly one of the first to popularize the lipid hy-pothesis. It is said that these ideas were spawned by what was perceived as counterintuitive information. He noted that North American busi-nessmen, among the most prosperous, nutritionally and financially, also were having markedly increased rates of heart disease. In post-war Europe, however, in the wake of reduced food supplies, heart disease was decreasing. He hypothesized that there was a connection between the amount and type of fat in the diet and the level of cholesterol in the blood and that this was further *correlated* with the development of heart diseases. He first published his suspicions of these correlations in *Circulation* magazine in 1963 (6). To give even greater credence to his hypothesis, he gathered diet and disease data from 22 countries for which this information was available at the time. For reasons that are not clear, he chose to analyze the data on only seven of the 22 coun-tries. These countries were: Italy, Greece, Finland, The Netherlands, the former Yugoslavia, Japan, and the USA. Using the data of these seven countries, he demonstrated a precise linear correlation between fat intake and cardiac death. Keys published his results in 1980. By the time I attended the School of Public Health in the late 80s, the study was frequently cited as groundbreaking and representing strong cor-relation, if not proof of the lipid hypothesis.

As mentioned above, one of the major weaknesses of observational studies is the presence of confounders, known and unknown. How can we be certain that diet — and specifically fat in the diet — is the main culprit in the development of heart disease and not other environmental factors or genetics? The Japanese migration studies are often cited as a creative way of clarifying this issue (7). A number of Japanese first migrated to the United States, primarily in what is now Hawaii and San Francisco, in the late 1800s to become part of the labor force (8). To this day, the largest concentration of Japanese-American citizens resides in these two areas. A group of investigators measured the blood cholesterol levels and heart attack rates of Japanese individuals in Japan, Hawaii and San Francisco. Those who settled in Hawaii had higher cholesterol levels and heart attack rates. The blood levels and attack rates were even more striking in the San Francisco immigrants. Since genetic changes can take several generations to manifest, it was reasonably hypothesized that the changes noted were due to environmental factors such as diet. The saturated fat content of the average diet in Hawaii and San Francisco was higher than that in Japan. Another point was scored for the lipid hypothesis.

The Framingham study is probably the oldest and most revered epidemiological investigation in the USA, if not the world (9). Over 1,000 papers have been published based on its findings. It was initiated in 1950 — and is still on going — in Framingham, Massachusetts. The original study group included 5,209 white men and women, representing about 25% of the town's population, between the ages of 30 to 62. At the outset, determinations were made of most of the known potential risk factors for heart disease, including blood cholesterol, blood pressure, diabetes, obesity, smoking habits and family history. Over the succeeding years, additional factors were added as more was learned about coronary artery disease. To the proponents of the lipid hypothesis, the cumulative findings of the Framingham Study over the past 60 years, provided, in the words of Steinberg, "the first solid and unarguable evidence that individuals with higher blood cholesterol levels at the time of the baseline examination were more likely to experience myocardial infarction in the subsequent years of follow up" (10). Furthermore, the findings were interpreted to show that cardiac risk factors were additive, that is, the risk of heart disease was greater for those with two or more risk factors. Therefore, this landmark epidemiological or observational study seemed to clearly demonstrate an association or *correlation* between blood cholesterol and heart disease, but did not prove *causality*. This would require an intervention study, an experiment, which is the classic hallmark of any true scientific endeavor, a clinical trial.

In keeping with the requirements of the scientific method, the clinical corollary of the "experiment" is the intervention trial. When we conduct an observational study, we recruit, for example, two groups; one has the exposure or risk factor of interest — smoking, obesity, hypertension, *etc.* — and the other group does not. We then follow them over time to determine which individuals develop the outcome of interest, heart disease, for example. However, we are not providing a treatment or intervention. In the clinical trial, we again recruit two groups — one for whom we provide the intervention such as a diet or drug suspected of affecting the outcome of interest — and the other group who does not receive the intervention. We follow both groups over time and determine what, if any, difference in outcome is found.

Numerous clinical trials conducted since the 1950s have attempted to answer the question as to what is the effect of the level and type of cholesterol in the blood on the development of heart disease and death from cardiac and non-cardiac causes. Most of the studies have been deemed flawed in some significant way; their results could be explained by chance alone and not due to the intervention because of too small a sample size or lacking in statistical significance. I will briefly mention only four of these studies.

In 1970, Paul Leren, a physician in Oslo, Norway, published the results of a 5-year study involving 412 survivors of heart attack (11). Half the group ate a diet high in polyunsaturated fats (largely from vegetable sources) and the other half continued on the typical Norwegian diet, which included higher saturated fat content such as meat, eggs, and cheese. At the end of the study period, 26% of those on the usual higher fat diet had a second heart attack compared to 16% in the group on the polyunsaturated fat diet. One of the criticisms of the study was that there was no difference in all-cause mortality, *i.e.* the group who ate less saturated fat may have just died from other non-cardiac causes, because the overall death rate was the same in the two groups.

In 1972, the result of the Finnish Mental Hospitals Study was published (12). Over 2,000 men and women in 2 hospitals were followed over a 12-year period. The patients in one hospital received a polyunsaturated-rich diet and the patients at the other hospital received the typical Finnish diet. The male patients in the experimental group experienced a 50% reduction in death from heart disease. The female patients also experienced a statistically significant reduction but to a lesser extent.

The Coronary Primary Prevention Trial (CPPT) (13) funded by the U.S. government involved 3,806 men between the ages of 35–59 followed for an average of 7.4 years. The treated group was given a powdered substance, cholestyramine, which is stirred into a liquid. This drug is a bile-binding agent, meaning that it works by binding the cholesterol which is excreted in the stool. The control group was reportedly given an equally unpleasant placebo. Those in the treatment group experienced only a 13.4 % reduction in total cholesterol, a 20% decrease in LDL or "bad" cholesterol and a 19% reduction in coronary events that was barely statistically significant. As a result of this trial the lipid hypothesis was more widely accepted and most of us began monitoring and treating high blood cholesterol. The trial was started in 1971, but the results were not available until 1984.

Cholestyramine was never a very popular drug because of its taste and lack of efficacy in terms of lowering the cholesterol numbers. With the discovery and marketing of the statins in the 1980s, the powdered substance was soon used only in the small group of patients who either refused to take statins or in whom there was some demonstrated side effect — an elevation in liver function tests or development of muscle pain or an elevation of muscle enzymes — as determined by blood tests.

In 2003, the results of ASCOT-LLA (Anglo-Scandinavian Cardiac Outcomes - Lipid Lowering Arm) trial was published (14). The very popular statin drug, Lipitor® ($12 billion in sales in 2008) was the treatment used. After 3.3 years of follow–up, the group reported a statistically significant 36% reduction in fatal and non-fatal heart attacks. At the end of an 8-year extension of the trial in 2011, ASCOT-LLA reported a 14% reduction in death from any cause. It has now reached the point where those who still challenge the lipid hypothesis or the efficacy of statins are regarded with pity, if not contempt. Skeptics remain, however, and their reservations are to follow.

The International Network of Cholesterol Skeptics (THINCS) is a group, to date, of approximately 100 researchers — MDs, PhDs, and science writers that are from all over the world, but primarily from Europe. According to its mission statement, "members of this group represent different views about the causation of atherosclerosis and cardiovascular disease…what we all oppose is that animal fat and high cholesterol play a role" (15). Daniel Steinberg in *The Cholesterol Wars*, acknowledges that skeptics do, in fact, exist, but he implies that they have been rightfully marginalized (16). He doesn't address the specific reservations of the doubters, but mentions them only in a general way in the appendix to his book in a section entitled "Frequently cited criticisms." He cites a 1978 survey of scientists working on some aspect of atherosclerosis research who were asked if they accepted that cholesterol was connected to coronary heart disease. Of the 189 who responded, 185 said yes, 2 were uncertain and 2 said no. Steinberg concludes with, "now that the statin results are in, the (lipid) hypothesis is established beyond doubt " (17). The identity of the 2 scientists who said no in the above survey is not known, but two of the long time skeptics and members of THINCS are Scottish physician, Malcolm Kendrick, author of *The Great Cholesterol Con* and Danish physician, researcher and spokesman for THINCS, Uffe Ravnskov, who has reportedly authored over 100 papers critical of the hypothesis and at least two books with which I am intimately familiar.

Unlike humans, whose diets consists of plant and animal products, the animals that have been studied and most famously reported on (Anitschow's rabbits) are vegetarians that lack the mechanism to process and break down dietary cholesterol and therefore when they are essentially force-fed a diet that is unnatural to them, their blood cholesterol levels rise extraordinarily high, which is not the case in human beings (18). It is generally appreciated that meat-eating humans and particularly North Americans who eat a relatively high fat diet will not likely raise their blood cholesterol levels by so much, even if they binge on meats, cheese, and eggs. In humans there appears to be a saturation principle. For example, let's say that you have a cholesterol level in the range of 225–250, like many Americans and you "pig out over the holidays" eating more high fat foods than usual. You will very likely raise your blood cholesterol level to perhaps, 275–300, but not 500–600, as would the forced-fed vegetarian rabbit or other herbivores. When an animal is forced to consume a diet that is unnatural for them, it is known that their blood cholesterol levels rise to levels unheard of in humans unless they have some underlying lipid disorder, familial hyperlipidemia, for example. Therefore, most skeptics, including Ravnskov and Kendrick, deny the relevance of these animal studies; they state that the disease artificially produced in animals cannot be reliably extrapolated to naturally living and eating human beings. Therefore, they consider the animal data to be irrelevant with respect to the development of human disease.

When the proponents of the lipid hypothesis offer genetic evidence for the hypothesis they frequently cite the example of familial hyperlipidemia (FH). There are 2 types of FH; the homozygous form arises when both parents have the condition and the heterozygous variant may be born when only one parent is affected. The former is quite rare, occurring in one in 1 million births and the latter, one in approximately 500 births. All of the cells in our body have the ability to take up cholesterol from the blood if their own production is inadequate. As mentioned previously, the apparatus on the surface of the cell that allows this uptake of cholesterol is the LDL receptor. People who are born with FH have a malfunctioning LDL receptor and therefore, less cholesterol is taken up into their cells, more remains in the blood and typically, these individuals have much higher cholesterol levels than the rest of us. The proponents argue that prior to the age of statins, FH patients were more likely to develop and die from coronary disease. The fact that everyone concedes that statins are extremely effective in lowering cholesterol numbers is offered as proof that cholesterol is the culprit and subduing the cause prevents disease and saves lives. The opponents of this hypothesis argue that FH patients not only inherit a defective LDL receptor, but they also have abnormally high levels of fibrinogen, Factor VIII, and prothrombin, which are all vital players in the body's blood clotting mechanisms (19). If we have too little of these factors, we can bleed too easily and if too much, the blood clots more readily, putting one at greater risk for a heart attack. In addition to lowering cholesterol, statins are known to have anti-clotting as well as anti-inflammatory properties, which the skeptics maintain more likely explains the positive effects of statins in FH patients.

As previously noted, the epidemiological evidence is the most controversial and often challenged. Ancel Keyes, while being credited for his "landmark" seven countries study is also most criticized by those who asked the reasonable question, "why did he choose to analyze the results from those particular countries and not any of the 15 others for which dietary information was available?" Could it be that those results confirmed what he believed to be the connection between diet and heart disease? Malcolm Kendrick states that had he chosen another seven — including France, Germany, Israel, Sweden, Switzerland, in addition to Finland and the Netherlands, he would have gotten completely opposite results (20). Kendrick then goes on to cite several additional studies including the Malmo-Sweden study of 2005 (21) and the Women's Health Initiative Study of 2006 (22), both large studies — 28,000 in the former and 48,000 in the latter — that followed subjects over a 6–8 year period and in neither was there a significant correlation between diet and stroke or cardiac deaths.

Ravnskov cites 15 studies (23) that refute the claim that high cholesterol is a cardiac risk factor for diabetic patients. In graduate school, I heard much about the so-called "French Paradox", the phenomenon of the French population having less cardiac disease and resulting death despite their higher saturated fat diet, than North Americans. The greater ingestion of red wine, with its alleged cardiac protective properties has been offered to explain this phenomenon. The critics of the lipid hypothesis then ask, how do we explain the "paradox" of the Maori, Massai or Polynesian people, all of whom consume a diet notoriously high in saturated fats yet they have only a fraction of the incidence of coronary disease (24), The critics argue that there is *no* paradox; cholesterol is simply not the culprit.

The basic argument against citing trial data in support of the lipid hypothesis is that the vast majority of studies demonstrate no response to the intervention (25-27) or that the positive effects are exaggerated or that the data were overly extrapolated.

So where does that leave us? What is the actual cause of heart disease, specifically, coronary heart disease that results in heart attacks? Not even the proponents of the lipid hypothesis maintain that high blood cholesterol is the only cause. It is generally appreciated or suspected that the causes of this disease are what is called multifactorial.

Virtually everyone acknowledges the role that smoking, hypertension, obesity, and diabetes play. The difference is that the proponents of the hypothesis believe, in the words of Daniel Steinberg, that high cholesterol in the blood is a "determining factor in the development of atherosclerosis and coronary heart disease and that correcting it would significantly reduce the burden of disease and its clinical consequences." The opponents believe that it is not only not *the* determining factor, but also not a factor at all. The opponents contend that the real culprit (s) are infection, inflammation and stress (28).

By stress, they are speaking not simply about the emotional stress that is associated with anxiety or a constantly worried-filled life. The mechanism is actually a bit more complicated involving the HPA system (29), which stands for Hypothalamic-Pituitary-Adrenal Axis. This is a very complex system or network involving the brain and the adrenal glands, which are located above the kidneys and, among other things, control how our bodies react to stress, regulate our moods, digestion and immune system. Proponents of the "stress hypothesis" often quote the results of the Interheart study, the results of which were published in the British medical magazine, *The Lancet* (30). The study involved over 30,000 patients participating at 232 centers in 52 countries throughout Africa, Asia, Europe, Latin and North America. The study identified 9 risk factors including psychosocial stress, which the authors stated accounts for over 90% of the risk for heart attack. The authors found that these factors were essentially the same for every racial or ethnic group, men and women, and in every geographic region in the world. For those of us who have always been champions of lifestyle modification, the results were encouraging and it was a wonderful breath of fresh air to see a large study without the Eurocentric preoccupation that is the basis of most of our "universal" recommendations in contemporary medicine. However, once again, we can regard the Interheart findings as, at best, suggestive, because of the nature of the study.

As previously mentioned, unlike experiments or trials, observational studies can only establish correlation between risk factors and outcome, not causality. The Interheart study was a particular type of observational study known as a cross-sectional or prevalence study — essentially a survey in which the risk factors and the disease of interest are determined at the same time. So while this type of study provides very interesting correlations — food for thought — it cannot be used to "prove" the "stress hypothesis." Stress, unlike cholesterol, cannot be measured quantitatively and western-trained physicians tend to be unimpressed with that which cannot be x-rayed, biopsied, or determined in a sample of body fluids. Cholesterol can be assigned a number — low, high or normal. The numbers can be followed over time and the effects of drugs or other interventions on the number can be determined — not so with the emotions. Research that deals with emotions tends to be regarded as "soft," unlike the imagined precision of the randomized clinical trial. A later chapter says more about this imaginativeness. It therefore appears that the skeptic's arguments against concluding that cholesterol is a principal factor in the development of heart disease is much more compelling than their assertion that the main culprit is stress.

My own personal ambivalence regarding the importance, central or otherwise, of cholesterol exemplifies precisely why relying exclusively on the gold standard, the randomized clinical trial, is problematic. There is a wealth of evidence implicating cholesterol as the culprit, however, the skeptics also offer compelling counter arguments, if one would only read and listen to them. The reality is that, as with so many things, consensus usually carries the day. Proponents of the lipid hypothesis often take the position of not wanting to dignify their critics' reservations and so they simply acknowledge that they exist, but won't discuss their specific criticisms. Implicitly, the skeptics are dismissed and grouped with other "deniers" such as those who deny human involvement in climate change or who reject Darwinian notions of evolution and specifically natural selection.

I still treat some levels of high cholesterol with drugs because I have usually practiced among high-risk populations with multiple risk factors and I am frankly uneasy about a diabetic with significantly elevated total and bad (LDL) cholesterol. However, I am not convinced that everyone has to have total cholesterol below 200 or every diabetic has to have an LDL lower than 100 or 70 as current dogma dictates. If a person has no other risk factors, I am not inclined to treat all individuals with drugs even though I appreciate that they are likely to be more effective in lowering the numbers than any degree of lifestyle change that most people are likely to make.

There are also medical legal reasons why it is difficult for medical providers *not* to treat high cholesterol. Since the lipid hypothesis is so widely accepted — it is a "slam-dunk" — and if a patient develops a presumed complication where high cholesterol is considered to be one of the culprits (consensus medicine), the physician would not likely win in case of a lawsuit because as Steinberg suggests "there is a preponderance of evidence in favor of the hypothesis."

When it comes to statin-phobia, which has been written about extensively, at least in the lay press (31, 32); I rely as much or more on personal experience than reported horror stories. In over 30 years, I have only rarely had to stop the medication because of obvious, clearly documented adverse effects — marked elevation in liver or muscle tests. It is always difficult to know what to make of patient's subjective complaints such as muscle or joint pain since these complaints are nonspecific and sometimes may be influenced by the patient's knowledge that statins *may* cause muscle damage. Aspirin may also cause life-threatening bleeding but this also is fortunately rare compared to the numbers of aspirins ingested in this country.

I believe that heart disease *is* multifactorial, and that the older you are, the more you're likely to get it. In some respects, the "explosion" in heart disease may actually represent the triumph in modern medicine and public health measures over infectious disease that use to kill most of us. I am not obsessed with cholesterol but feel better if the numbers are low, rather than high and I have never reflexively treated "abnormal numbers." It depends on age, other risk factors, the patient's current quality of life and what they are willing to accept. It is an *individual* decision based upon a conversation with an individual man or woman.

References Cited

1. Steinberg, D., *The Cholesterol Wars: The Skeptics Vs. the Preponderance of Evidence*. Amsterdam: Academic Press. 2007. p.1.
2. Ibid. p.2.
3. Ibid. p.24.
4. Ibid. pp.28-29.
5. Wise, L.A., J.R. Palmer, D. Reich, Y.C. Cozier, and L. Rosenberg, Hair relaxer use and risk of uterine leiomyomata in African-American women. *American Journal of Epidemiology*, 2012. **175**(5): p. 432-440.
6. Keys, A., H.L. Taylor, H. Blackburn, J. Brozek, J.T. Anderson, and E. Simonson, Coronary heart disease among Minnesota business and professional men followed fifteen years. *Circulation*, 1963. **28**(3): p. 381-395.
7. Marmot, M., S. Syme, A. Kagan, H. Kato, J. Cohen, and J. Belsky, Epidemiologic studies of coronary heart disease and stroke in Japanese men living in Japan, Hawaii and California: prevalence of coronary and hypertensive heart disease and associated risk factors. *American Journal of Epidemiology*, 1975. **102**(6): p. 514-525.
8. *Immigration, The Journey to American: The Japanese*. [cited 2013 September 1]; Available from: http://library.thinkquest.org/20619/Japanese.html.
9. *History of the Framingham Heart Study*. [cited 2013 September 1];

Available from: http://www.framinghamheartstudy.org/about/history.html.

10. Steinberg, D. p. 36.

11. Leren, P., The Oslo diet-heart study eleven-year report. *Circulation*, 1970. **42**(5): p. 935-942.

12. Miettinen, M., M. Karvonen, O. Turpeinen, R. Elosuo, and E. Paavilainen, Effect of cholesterol-lowering diet on mortality from coronary heart-disease and other causes: a twelve-year clinical trial in men and women. *The Lancet*, 1972. **300**(7782): p. 835-838.

13. The Lipid Research Clinics Coronary Primary Prevention Trial results. I. Reduction in incidence of coronary heart disease. *JAMA*, 1984. **251**(3): p. 351-64.

14. Sever, P.S., B. Dahlöf, N.R. Poulter, H. Wedel, G. Beevers, M. Caulfield, R. Collins, S.E. Kjeldsen, A. Kristinsson, and G.T. McInnes, Prevention of coronary and stroke events with atorvastatin in hypertensive patients who have average or lower-than-average cholesterol concentrations, in the Anglo-Scandinavian Cardiac Outcomes Trial—Lipid Lowering Arm (ASCOT-LLA): a multicentre randomised controlled trial. *The Lancet*, 2003. **361**(9364): p. 1149-1158.

15. *The International Network of Cholesterol Skeptics.* [cited 2013 September 2]; Available from: http://www.thincs.org/.

16. Steinberg, D. p.211.

17. Ibid.

18. Ravnskov, U., The Cholesterol Myths: Exposing the Fallacy that Saturated Fat and Cholesterol Cause Heart Disease. Washington, D.C.: New Trends Pub., 2000. p.139.

19. Kendrick, M., The Great Cholesterol Con: The Truth About What Really Causes Heart Disease and How to Avoid It. London: John Blake, 2007. p. 231.

20. Ibid. p.53-56.

21. Leosdottir, M., P. Nilsson, J.Å. NILSSON, H. Månsson, and G.

Berglund, Dietary fat intake and early mortality patterns–data from The Malmö Diet and Cancer Study. *Journal of Internal Medicine*, 2005. **258**(2): p. 153-165.

22. Howard, B.V., L. Van Horn, J. Hsia, J.E. Manson, M.L. Stefanick, S. Wassertheil-Smoller, L.H. Kuller, A.Z. LaCroix, R.D. Langer, and N.L. Lasser, Low-fat dietary pattern and risk of cardiovascular disease. *JAMA*. 2006. **295**(6): p. 655-666.

23. Ravnskov, U. p.62.

24. Petersen, I.B. *The Massai keep healthy despite a high-fat diet*. 2012 [cited 2013 August 28]; Available from: http://sciencenordic.com/maasai-keep-healthy-despite-high-fat-diet.

25. Ravnskov, U., *Ignore the Awkward! How the Cholesterol Myths are Kept Alive*. Charleston, SC: CreateSpace, 2010. p. 154.

26. Ravnskov, U., *Ignore the Awkward!* pp. 133-135.

27. Kendrick, M. pp.237-252.

28. Colpo, A., The Great Cholesterol Con. Why Everything You've been Told About Cholesterol, Diet and Heart Disease is Wrong. London: John Blake Publishing Ltd., 2006. pp.134-148.

29. Randall, M. *The Physiology of Stress: Cortisol and the Hypothalamic-Pituitary- Adrenal Axis*. 2011 [cited 2013 July 21]; Available from: http://dujs.dartmouth.edu/fall-2010/the-physiology-of-stress-cortisol-and-the-hypothalamic-pituitary-adrenal-axis - .UjXmWLzFavk.

30. Yusuf, S., S. Hawken, S. Ôunpuu, T. Dans, A. Avezum, F. Lanas, M. McQueen, A. Budaj, P. Pais, and J. Varigos, Effect of potentially modifiable risk factors associated with myocardial infarction in 52 countries (the INTERHEART study): case-control study. *The Lancet*, 2004. **364**(9438): p. 937-952.

31. Colpo A. 2006.

32 Graveline, D. *Statin Drugs Side Effects: The Misguided War on Cholesterol*. United States: Duane Graveline, 2006.

CHAPTER 9

What About Alternative Medicine?

THROUGHOUT THE PRECEDING pages, my emphasis has been on what is commonly referred to as conventional, orthodox, or allopathic medicine. This represents the dominant medical paradigm in this country and much of the western world. The major therapeutic modalities include drugs manufactured and promoted by pharmaceutical companies, surgery, and radiation therapy — particularly in the treatment of various cancers.

The orthodox medical community has alienated a large segment of the population because many of its treatments are perceived of as being too expensive, ineffective, and having an unacceptably high level of side effects. The FDA, whose role it is to ensure the safety of food and drugs has had its credibility questioned in the recent past with the controversy regarding the approval and then banning of cholesterol lowering drugs and then anti-inflammatory medications used commonly for arthritis. In 1997, the FDA approved the cholesterol-lowering drug, Baycol (a statin). The manufacturer, Bayer, however, withdrew the drug after 4 years because 31 patients taking the medication died from a severe muscle disease called rhabdomyolysis. All statins have a similar mechanism of action, therefore concern was justifiable that all statins may produce similar side effects. Assurances were offered that, while all statins can have an effect on muscle tissue, Baycol was felt to be particularly toxic. Also the 31 individuals who died were either taking other medications that were especially dangerous in combination with Baycol or were taking a much higher initial dose than was recommended. Many remained unconvinced and several books have been written chronicling the potential and real dangers of statins (1-3). In 2004, Merck & Co. pulled Vioxx off the market because Vioxx was found to be associated with an increased risk of heart attacks and stroke. The following year, the FDA asked Pfizer to remove its anti-inflammatory, Bextra, from the market because the risks of heart disease, stroke, and skin complications — namely a severe blistering and sloughing of the skin known as Stevens-Johnson Syndrome — was found to outweigh the drug's benefits. For all that its worth, it is noteworthy that Wikipedia lists 30 drugs that have been withdrawn in the US, Canada, and Europe since the year 2000 because of toxicity or lack of efficacy (4).

The term alternative or complementary medicine (hereafter referred to as CAM) has various definitions. As defined by David Eisenberg, author of an often-cited article published in the *New England Journal of Medicine* in 1993, CAM consists of "those medical interventions not taught widely at US medical schools or generally available at US hospitals (5)." It may also be referred to as those practices not part of the dominant medical system of a country and may include, but is not restricted to herbal medicine, acupuncture, homeopathy, chiropractic, and the use of megadose — far exceeding the official daily recommended amounts — vitamin therapy.

Herbal medicine or more specifically "traditional Chinese medicine, reportedly focuses on restoring a balance of energy, body and spirit to maintain health rather than treating a particular disease or medical condition" (6). Over the years, I have had several patients and relatives who told me that they were taking some "Chinese herbs," but had little knowledge of the precise contents. This is understandable because typically a variety of herbs are used such as green tea, gingko, ginseng, astragals, and others. It is said that, in China, "more than 3200 herbs and 300 mineral and animal extracts are used in more than 400 different formulas; various formulas may contain anywhere from 4 to 12 different ingredients which are then taken in the form of teas, powders or pills" (7). Various cultures all over the world have used herbs to maintain health and treat specific diseases. "Chinese herbal medicine developed as part of its culture from tribal roots and by 200 years before the Christian era, traditional Chinese medicine was firmly established" (8).

Acupuncture is another remedy of eastern origin. For those of us who were trained in orthodox medical schools and studied western concepts of anatomy and physiology, the principles behind acupuncture are difficult to understand. To even begin to make sense of the rationale, however, it is important to try to understand the traditional Chinese philosophy upon which acupuncture is based. The philosophy maintains that an energy flow exists in every living being that is necessary for life. This energy force is called "Chi" (pronounced chee). This energy is said to flow through the body in channels called acupuncture meridians. Each meridian controls or influences an organ, with different meridians for the heart, lung, liver, *etc.* In the healthy person the Chi flows through all the channels smoothly. Obstructed energy flow leads to sickness. An acupuncture point is a specific area on the skin that reflects a disturbance in a particular organ. By placing tiny needles in these points, the obstruction can be cleared and contribute to healing. This is, of course, a gross oversimplification, but probably adequate for my intent in this chapter. For those who wish to go much deeper, there is an older text by Toguchi and Warren (9) and several other introductory papers online.

Most of us in the US are far more familiar with chiropractics — often considered another modality of CAM — that has long been used as a common pain relief for acute and chronic pain syndromes involving muscles, joints, connective tissues, and bones. It traditionally is a manual spinal manipulation based upon the theory that proper alignment of the body's musculoskeletal system enables the body to heal itself without the use of drugs or surgery. One who visits a chiropractor will find that they take a medical history and perform a physical examination as does the allopath. They then perform various diagnostic procedures — namely x-rays — and then determine if treatment is appropriate (anecdotal perhaps, but as in all of medicine, it is almost always deemed appropriate). The treatment plan may involve one or more — almost always more — usually 2–3 treatments per week, or until you stop coming —manipulations. Treatments generally consist of manual adjustments in which the doctor manipulates the spine. Many chiropractors also incorporate nutritional counseling and exercise prescriptions.

Several other CAM modalities including reflexology, iridology, naturopathy, therapeutic touch, *etc.* However, a reasonable discussion of all of these interventions is beyond the scope of this chapter. Suffice it to say that most practitioners of orthodox medicine are convinced that they are in the category of "quack medicine" and the proponents of CAM generally consider all or most of them to be of value. I will provide my mild to moderately informed two cents at the end of this chapter.

As was suggested earlier, CAM is a rather large tent under which can be found various disciplines. Some of these approaches such as acupuncture and traditional Chinese herbal medicine have been practiced for thousands of years. The modern era of CAM, however received a major boost in the 1970s and 80s, probably due in part to a perceived growing depersonalization of orthodox medicine. This was likely triggered by the development of the HMOs, *i.e.* an increasing corporatization of medicine. I distinctly remember when the administration of a hospital with which I was affiliated in Harlem began referring to patients as "clients," and we were encouraged to limit office visits to 10–15 minutes. At another hospital where I worked in Queens, the "bottom line," — which could be calculated in terms of dollars and cents — was paramount, with less emphasis being placed on patient satisfaction.

The growing interest in CAM is not only due to the real and perceived failures of orthodoxy but also because of the sense of empowerment one gets from taking matters into one's own hands — in treating oneself rather than feeling at the mercy of often impersonal doctors and institutions. It also is likely that one of the main reasons for the acceptance of CAM is that some of these healthcare practices are more consistent with the values, beliefs, and philosophical attitudes toward health and life of many people. I have had countless patients tell me over the years, "Doc, I'm just not a pill person. Whenever we got sick, I remember my mother or grandmother preparing…." Granted, I have no doubt that patients have very selective memories and may imagine that grandmother or the nice family doctor who visited them in the home were able to perform extraordinary feats when nothing of the kind actually happened. Many of the conditions were likely self-limiting and would have gotten better irrespective of what was done. However, perception is everything and a poor memory goes a long way.

There are several major league proponents of CAM, particularly in the US, but some of the more familiar names are Deepak Chopra, Gary Null, Andrew Weil, and the newest kid on the block, Mehmet (Dr.) Oz.

Chopra is an Indian born physician who immigrated to the US in 1970. He is board certified in internal medicine with a specialty in endocrinology — diabetes and thyroid diseases, for example. He worked in orthodox medicine for several years and reportedly met a noted doctor of Ayurvedic medicine in the 1980s. Ayurvedic comes from the

Sanskrit, Ayur (life) and Vedic (science or knowledge). It is one of the world's oldest healing traditions, having been used in India for up to five thousand years. According to Ayurveda, "human beings consist of 3 bodies or aspects: the body, mind and spirit. This system emphasizes that health is a harmonious functioning of all three parts of this trinity" (10). It is perceived as a practice that is both spiritual and practical. Its therapeutic modalities include diet, herbs, exercise, and meditation.

Chopra reportedly met the Guru Mahareshi Mahesh Yogi in 1985 who advised him to start an Ayurvedic Health Center, which he ultimately did. In the early 1990s he left orthodox medicine reportedly, at least in part, because of his disenchantment with having to prescribe too many drugs (11) — a sentiment with which I can most definitely relate. After the 1993 publication of his book, *Ageless Body, Timeless Mind,* he secured an interview on the Oprah ("Midas Touch") Winfrey show and he was off, ultimately starting the Chopra Center For Well Being in 1996. To date he has published anywhere from 35 to 65 books — the precise number is uncertain as several of them have not been translated into English. He is a literal CAM industry unto himself, being more on the mystical side.

Gary Null, the non-physician in this quartet of CAM heavyweights that I will briefly discuss, is a well known radio talk show host, lecturer, prolific writer of several (very large) books, and an exceedingly energetic promoter of numerous products on his website and public TV. He reportedly holds Ph.D.s in human nutrition and public health sciences. The legitimacy of his credentials have been questioned by self-styled "quackbuster" Stephen Barrett, M.D, a retired psychiatrist who seems to have devoted much of his life to rooting out what he perceives as fraud and chicanery in CAM. Barrett admits to "following Null's activities since the early 1970's"(12). I tend to be less impressed with academic credentials alone as, over the years, I have known a fair amount of fools who are Ivy League graduates, and sages who have not finished high school. Anyway, I listened to Null's radio program on the Pacifica station, WBAI in New York from 1986–2007. Many of his claims span the range of interesting to improbable to farfetched — nutritional formulas to grow "a healthy head of hair" in adulthood (after becoming bald) to "proven" dangers of fluoridation and mercury fillings, to his anti-immunization stance, to denying the role of HIV in AIDS. He is an extraordinarily articulate and well-versed proponent of his positions, and unless one is typically closed minded and dismissive, one often feels compelled to at least do their homework and take a look at some of what he says. As a very busy practitioner, I simple didn't have the time to investigate many of the unconventional ideas that he proposed; however, the primary value that he offers is good, common sense advice on the crucial role of lifestyle in gaining and maintaining health. I saw no downside to his message of following a healthy diet, exercising, and attempting to achieve "balance in one's life." This upside can be said about most, if not all CAM practitioners.

Mehmet (Dr.) Oz clearly has the strongest establishment credentials of all the current Gurus. He is a cardiothoracic (heart) surgeon, vice-chair and professor of surgery at New York Presbyterian. I remember when I first saw him at a conference in New York several years before the Oprah phenomenon. I was impressed and pleasantly surprised to hear this surgeon speaking about the importance of nutrition. Probably Oz's greatest public health potential is the fact that his message will more likely resonant with a wider audience because of his credentials, and TV program, of course. His words carry more weight than a nutritionist or a family doctor who may be saying the same things. Of course, as Lord Acton so famously said, "power tends to corrupt and absolute power tends to corrupt absolutely." Oz has gone from just giving sound lifestyle advice to promoting a range of products and gimmicks. Such endorsements include raspberry ketone and green coffee extract capsules, conjugated linoleic acid, and Garcinia Cambogia — alleged fat burners useful in rapid weight loss that are not always backed by rigorous scientific investigations. I am aware of one small (60 people), short

(8 weeks) study that was published in 2004 that suggested the value of Garcinia Cambogia in very modest weight loss (13). It must be said that many products use his name without his permission and that he reportedly does not benefit directly from product sales. According to a March, 2013 airing of Good Morning America, Oz was sued in 2012 by a 76 year old diabetic with neuropathy (nerve damage) who reportedly sustained severe burns of his feet after using one of Oz's suggested knapsack heated rice footsies to cure insomnia. Now, of course, any doctor who treats patients or gives advice runs the risk of being sued, but herein lies the danger of indirectly treating strangers over the radio or TV. On one of his programs, Oz admitted that his wife has treated their children with homeopathic remedies, which sounds at least somewhat like an endorsement. Homeopathic remedies "are generally dilutions of natural substances from plant, minerals and animals…the more dilute the remedy, the greater the potency," (14) so that seemingly only the essence of the substance remains. I admit, I don't know how this would work but if it does by whatever mechanism, then so be it. Oddly, Oz feels that we need to spend more time getting to know the quality of our stool. I don't know, how familiar? Other than solid or loose, brown or black or red — which could suggest bleeding — I'm not sure we need to get much more familiar.

I think it was Horace Greeley who said that there is a sucker born every minute. If he was just speaking of Americans, I think he was overly optimistic. Dr. Oz has a huge stage upon which he can, and has I suspect, made a major public health contribution. It seems that it is therefore incumbent upon him to be a bit more mindful of his comments. He speaks so glowingly of the value of science that one would think that he would want to be on more solid footing before making comments and recommendations to millions, especially in a country that has such a problem with obesity and an obsession with quick weight loss schemes.

Perhaps the father of the modern CAM movement is Andrew Weil, a graduate of Harvard College and its medical school. Shortly after just completing 1 post-graduate year in orthodox medicine, he became a drug researcher (he was a botany major at Harvard undergraduate school) and then launched a very successful writing career with the publication of his first book, *The Natural Mind* in 1972. This is a very significant book for the CAM movement because it laid the foundation and at least popularized the intellectual precepts of the movement. Weil advises a greater reliance on intuition than on what he terms "mere intellection." He says, "there exists within us a source of direct information about reality that can teach us all we need to know" (15). He continues "we live in an infinite universe where everything is relative" (16). So it's not all about the scientific method. Weil believes that "the power to heal, like the power to make ill, resides in the patient" (17). He gives credence to faith healing, stating "it is held in contempt by most rational people, despite the abundant evidence of cures"(18). As is the case with too many CAM promoters, however, he fails to illustrate any of this abundance of evidence. Like the other members of the quartet previously discussed, he is not an extraordinary and effective spokesperson by accident. He is an engaging writer and speaker, articulate, and on so many levels makes so much sense. He talks about wanting to see a coordination and ultimate synthesis of the intuition of ancient medicine with the intellection of modern western medicine. He too speaks often of being balanced. On a personal level, he seems to be a nice enough guy, having been helpful to me when I met him at a CAM conference in the 90s when he gave me some useful advice on what to do for my wife's sinus problems; "stinging nettle" which worked for a while — as do many things for a while. He has also appeared on the Oprah show a few times and in 1997 and 2005 he appeared on the cover of Time magazine. The desire for openness and synthesis of various ways of healing is laudable, but the glib statements of opinion and wishful thinking is problematic. Weil states,

Since leaving the world of allopathic practice, I have witnessed a number of impressive non allopathic cures of serious allergies, infections, and toxic reactions. I have also studied reliable reports from colleagues and friends of non-allopathic cures of more dramatic diseases, including cancer and life threatening infections (19).

Well maybe, but where is the evidence for any of this? This sounds like all too typical CAM hyperbole.

The fundamental criticism of CAM from allopathic or orthodox practitioners is that it is unscientific, not evidenced-based. It is charged that the claims are based primarily on anecdotes and testimonials rather than trial data. This is generally true, however, in 1997, Gary Null published an approximately 900 page book that was touted as the first comprehensive guide to scientific peer review studies of natural supplements and their proven treatment values(20). The book contains numerous citations of studies, although the descriptions and interpretations are provided by Null and one would have to do some serious investigation to determine the validity of his conclusions. It is for this reason that I would be reluctant to dismiss the referenced findings. I am not aware that Null's critics even take the time to evaluate his "data." As he is less visible than the other members of the quartet, he is rarely mentioned in critiques of CAM. Stephen Barrett, of Quackwatch, seems to be the only critic paying much attention, virtually bordering on obsession.

A major criticism of CAM is typified in the statement of Paul Kurtz, publisher of the *Scientific Review of Alternative Medicine*, "the uncritical public acceptance of health fads and diets can be dangerous to the public's health, especially if people substitute these nostrums for competent medical treatment"(21). There are situations where this can be a legitimate source of concern. For example, in the 1990s, Burton Goldberg, entrepreneur and compiler of the *Alternative Medicine- The Definitive Guide*, touted cancer treatments offered in Mexico (22), that even Gary Null criticized as taking advantage of desperate cancer patients who were required to pay several thousands of dollars for questionable treatments. If, in fact, people are duped into substituting "proven" treatments for expensive, unproven, and especially ineffective therapies then this is a cause for concern. However, critics often assume that the definition of proven means tested in randomized trials and subsequently approved by the FDA.

I would remind you of the number of the drugs that have been recalled for lack of efficacy or toxicity that were thought to represent proven treatments. It has been estimated that approximately 100 thousand Americans die each year from prescription drugs (23). Suppose this figure is a gross exaggeration. Suppose only 50 thousand die from FDA approved drugs. Would that be more tolerable? In 1999, the Institute of Medicine reported that up to 98 thousand people die each year because of mistakes in hospitals. The figure was updated to at least 210 thousand in 2010 (24). Keep in mind that the hospital is generally considered the great bastion of "competent allopathic treatment." Could you imagine the orthodox outrage and sense of horror that would be generated if even a tiny fraction of that number of deaths could be proven to be due to CAM treatments?

As a practitioner of essentially orthodox internal medicine over the years, I have found myself prescribing a whole host of "nostrums" which have been proven to be effective in clinical trials but resoundingly ineffective in practice — various anti-inflammatory medications, drugs for neuropathy (nerve pain), abdominal pain due to acid reflux, and a host of others. Despite the frequent lack of efficacy and occasional toxicity, they are not dismissed as quack remedies. In an essay on Alternative Medicine and the Psychology of Belief (25), psychologist Joseph Alcock stated that medical science must determine what constitutes a real effective rate as opposed to an apparent effective rate of a given medicine. He seems to find it troubling that a person may improve "whether the medicine is helpful or not." I think, however, that patients are primarily concerned with outcomes and are not especially troubled by the fact that the placebo effect may be playing a role. A placebo is an inert substance, one that does not cause a physical change but is perceived as having one. Particularly with pain syndromes, the goal is to feel better, and if the placebo effect can be "harnessed" as Andrew Weil has suggested, nothing is wrong with that.

My anecdotal observations over the years is that most supplements and herbs as commonly taken by most patients are harmless and probably ineffective in terms of what they are touted to accomplish. I have admittedly ambivalent but evolving opinions on the issue of regulation. Based upon the definition of a drug in the Food, Drug and Cosmetic Act of 1938, many of these CAM treatments would appear to, in fact, be "substances intended for use in the diagnosis, cure, mitigation, treatment or prevention of disease." Furthermore, many are "substances other than food intended to affect the structure or function of the body (26)." It would seem that if a substance is deemed to be effective, is not just a placebo, and it meets the above criteria, then it is a drug and should be tested, monitored, and regulated, all in the interest of public safety. With the enactment of the Dietary-Supplement Health and Education Act (DSHEA) in 1994, herbal remedies, for example were allowed to be sold without the manufactures being required to prove their effectiveness and safety to the FDA (27). As an indication of my ambivalence, however, as long as the labeling of these products continue to include the statement that the product has not been evaluated by the FDA or that efficacy has not been demonstrated in clinical trials, then "buyer beware." If the potential customer is made aware of the above and chooses to purchase and use it, this should be their prerogative. I would reject the paternalism implied in trying to protect people from themselves unless the dangers have been demonstrated and are clear.

Studies of various CAM techniques such as acupuncture and Chinese herbal medicine may never be able to be conducted to the satisfaction of those who place their unremitting trust in the randomized clinical trial (RCT). Therefore the claims of CAM proponents will not likely be substantiated to the extent required by CAM skeptics and so what? As I suggested in the chapter on universal vaccinations, it ultimately breaks down to the role of personal responsibility. Even given the rigors of the RCT, doctors have been labelled the "3rd leading cause of death" in this country, due to the prescription drugs and hospital deaths (28). People it seems, especially Americans, are an extraordinarily gullible bunch and there may be no way of saving them from themselves.

The politically correct statement, "first talk to your doctor or pharmacist before using any of these products" is frequently used in the literature of CAM proponents and also by orthodox organizations such as the American Cancer Society. The reality is, however, that most doctors and pharmacists know little about these products. In the ideal world, CAM products and techniques would be studied in schools of medicine and pharmacy, *especially if studies have found them to be efficacious and safe*. Rather than being abolished, as suggested by some CAM critics (29), the National Center For Complementary and Alternative Medicine (NCCAM) should receive even greater funding. There are promising trends. The Office of Alternative Medicine was established by the US Congress in 1992 under the National Institutes of Health and received 2 million dollars in funding initially. Today it has been expanded to an independent agency, the National Center For Complementary and Alternative Medicine (NCCAM) and now receives 87 million in funding. Many consider this a waste of taxpayer money, but I don't hear equal outrage at the millions that go to waste on military spending in general and armaments never to be used in particular, but that's another book. What price public health?

Irrespective of what we are taught in the universities, providers of medicine should want to expand their knowledge base to include CAM. Since Americans spent (out of pocket) 34 billion dollars on CAM in 2009 (30), there is evidence that the field is at least stable if not growing. As money drives much of what we do in this country, the competition to orthodox medicine may become so fierce that American medical education may be forced to take a closer look and incorporate at least some aspects of CAM in the curricula of professional schools.

Given our current state of knowledge, despite the very serious and real concerns that one may justifiably have with orthodox medicine, it would behoove the prospective consumer or patient to be equally wary of the practitioners of CAM and their treatments. The orthodox and CAM communities, especially the leadership, have more in common than they are both prepared to concede. The messages are often based on engendering fear in the prospective customers and ignorance or lack of information is a key ingredient in ensuring their continued success. The arrogance of orthodoxy is typified in a statement made by 2 editors in the *Journal of the American Medical Association* (JAMA) in 1998, "there is no alternative medicine, only scientifically proven evidence-based medicine supported by solid data OR unproven medicine for which scientific evidence is lacking" (31). The orthodox scientific community (at least those published in the more prestigious trade journals such as *The New England Journal of Medicine, Annals* or, *Archives of Internal Medicine* seem to usually come to the conclusion that ultimately we need to take more pharmaceuticals. The criteria for unacceptably high cholesterol, blood sugar, or blood pressure continue to be updated in a way that increases several-fold the number of persons requiring medication. As the perception or definition of normal changes, it becomes increasingly apparent that most of us will eventually have to take drugs to satisfy these criteria for normal pressure, sugar, or cholesterol. Fortunately for the pharmaceutical industry, it is recognized that few people will make the dramatic lifestyle changes often necessary to normalize these numbers by so-called natural means. On the CAM side, if you listen to some of these gurus, you will be told that despite what you may have believed, you, most of us, perhaps 95% of the population is really sick and don't realize it. If you go to the doctor for a check up and are given a clean bill of health, the probability is, they would say, the doctor didn't run the proper tests to reveal the diseases, allergies, *etc.* that you invariably have. I have had several patients coming to the office requesting saliva or hair analysis based upon what they read online or heard on TV. Often these online or TV gurus will have the answers to yours and everyone else's health problems if you purchase their books and unending products; products which are touted to treat, if not cure, literally everything from AIDS to xerosis (dry skin). You will often see their informercials on cable TV or hear them on one of a number of radio programs on AM or FM. If you visit most health food stores (where I have lived in New York City or Atlanta, anyway) you will often see ill-informed salespersons giving self-serving medical advice to the equally ill-informed; many looking for remedies for anything from hypertension, diabetes, to erectile dysfunction, or constipation. Like many con artists, these salespersons, wherever they operate, begin with a premise that is very reasonable. They claim that the orthodox medical system is sick, and in need of repair and often makes people sick. They then proceed to exaggerate to produce fear and profit. They do often take advantage of desperate people and the general population by trying to convince them that virtually every disease, in any stage, or any condition is preventable or curable. They would have you believe that the first step to your cure is to buy whatever they are selling and the pressure is then applied to get you to continue buying.

The point of this section is to alert readers to the fact that both camps have much to offer and deserve to be looked at seriously; however, recognize that they are like two armed camps competing for the minds and pocketbooks of the masses of the people. Both self-righteously claim to care only about the public health, and both are multibillion dollar a year industries. I do not mean to imply a false equivalency here. In the words of the late Canadian psychology professor, Barry Beyerstein, "*scientific biomedicine* (italics mine), unlike CAM is institutionally committed to finding empirical support for its treatments and eventually weeds out those that fail to pass the muster" (32).

From 1991 to 1997 alone, total American visits to CAM practitioners increased from 427 to 629 million (33). As noted, almost 35 billion is spent on CAM each year — in spite of the deep pockets of orthodox medicine that is well known in its capacity to effectively lobby Congress. As I have advised my patients over the years, your body, your mind, and your health is much too valuable to be passively given over entirely to strangers, be they M.D.s, herbalists, radio, TV gurus, or any other experts. Question, investigate, and take nothing for granted. Trusts your instincts, but not unconditionally.

References Cited

1. Graveline, D., *Statin Drugs Side Effects and the Misguided War on Cholesterol*. 2006, United States: Duane Graveline

2. Graveline, D., *The Dark Side of Statins*, 2010, Duane Graveline.

3. Roberts, B.H., *The Truth about Statins : Risks and Alternatives to Cholesterol-Lowering Drugs*. 2012, New York: Gallery Books.

4. List of withdrawn drugs. [cited 2013 November 12]; Available from: http://en.wikipedia.org/wiki/List_of_withdrawn_drugs.

5. Eisenberg, D.M., R.C. Kessler, C. Foster, F.E. Norlock, D.R. Calkins, and T.L. Delbanco, Unconventional medicine in the United States--prevalence, costs, and patterns of use. New England Journal of Medicine, 1993. **328**(4): p. 246-252.

6. Chinese Herbal Medicine. 2011 [cited 2013 October 19]; Available from: http://www.cancer.org/treatment/treatment-sandsideeffects/complementaryandalternativemedicine/herbsvitaminsandminerals/chinese-herbal-medicine.

7. Ibid.

8. Ibid.

9. Gerson, S., *Ayurveda : The Ancient Indian Healing Art.* [New issue.]. ed. The health essentials series; Variation: Health essentials series. 1997, Shaftesbury, Dorset: Rockport, Mass. p.3

10. Ibid.

11. Boer, H.A., The Work of Andrew Weil and Deepak Chopra-Two Holistic Health/New Age Gurus: A Critique of the Holistic Health/New Age Movements. *Medical Anthropology Quarterly*, 2003. **17**(2): p. 233-250.

12. Barrett, S. A critical look at Gary Null's Activities and Credentials. 2012 [cited 2013 November 28]; Available from: http://www.quackwatch.com/04ConsumerEducation/null.html.

13. Heymsfield, S.B., L.J. Aronne, and G.L. Blackburn, HCA efficiency. *Diabetes, Obesity and Metabolism*, 2004. **6**(6): p. 458-459.

14. *Alternative medicine : The Definitive Guide.* 1993, Puyallup, WA: Future Medicine Pub. pp.272-274.

15. Weil, A., *The Natural Mind: A New Way of Looking at Drugs and the Higher Consciousness.* 1972: Boston: Houghton Mifflin. p. 152.

16. Ibid.

17. Ibid., p.168.

18. Ibid., p.171.

19. Ibid., p.169.

20. Null, G., *The Clinician's Handbook of Natural Healing.* 1998, New York: Kensington Books.

21. Kurtz, P. In defense of scientific medicine, in Sampson, W. and Lewis, V., eds. *Science Meets Alternative Medicine : What the Evidence Says About Unconventional Treatments*, 2000, Prometheus Books.

22. *Alternative Medicine : The Definitive Guide*, 1995, Puyallup, WA : Future Medicine Pub.

23. Starfield, B., Is US health really the best in the world? *Journal of the American Medical Association*, 2000. **284**(4): p. 483-485.

24. Allen, M.and Propublica. How many die from medical mistakes in U.S. hospitals. *Scientific American*, Sept. 20, 2013.

25. Alcock, J.E. Alternative medicine and the psycology of belief, in Sampson, W. and Lewis, V., eds. Science Meets Alternative Medicine : What the Evidence Says About Unconventional Treatments, 2000, Prometheus Books.`

26. FD&C Act Chapters I and II: Short Definitions. 2012 [cited 2013 September 15]; Available from: http://www.fda.gov/RegulatoryInformation/Legislation/FederalFoodDrugandCosmeticActFDCAct/FDCActChaptersIandIIShortTitleandDefinitions/ucm086297.htm.

27. Kutz, P. in *Science meets alternative medicine : what the evidence says about unconventional treatments*.

28. Starfield, B., *The Journal of the American Medical Association*, 2000. **284**(4): p. 483-485.

29. Mielczarek, E. V., and Engler, B. D. (2012). Measuring mythology: startling concepts in NCCAM grants. Skeptical Inquirer, 36, 36-43.

30. Nahin, R.L., *Costs of Complementary and Alternative Medicine (CAM) and Frequency of Visits to CAM Practitioners*: US 2007. 2010: DIANE Publishing

31. Fontanarosa, P.B. and G.D. Lundberg, Alternative medicine meets science. *Journal of the American Medical Association*, 1998. **280**(18): p. 1618-1619.

32. Beyerstein, B. Social and judgenmental biases that make inert treatments seem to work. in Sampson, W. and Lewis, V., eds. *Science Meets Alternative Medicine : What the Evidence Says About Unconventional Treatments*, 2000, Prometheus Books.

33. Eisenberg, D.M., R.C. Kessler, C. Foster, F.E. Norlock, D.R. Calkins, and T.L. Delbanco, Unconventional medicine in the United States--prevalence, costs, and patterns of use. *New England Journal of Medicine*, 1993. **328**(4): p. 246-252.

CHAPTER 10

The Delusion of Certainty

TO LIVE WITH uncertainty can be, at best, anxiety-provoking and, at worst, paralyzing. This desire, for certainty accounts, in some part, I suspect, for the very human need for some form of religion. For religion is, among other things, an attempt to explain the inexplicable, to provide answers where there are none. There are many who haughtily dismiss religion, but at the same time, embrace scientism, which for our purposes may be defined as a dogmatic belief in the universal applicability of the scientific method to reduce all of knowledge to a measureable entity. Both in terms of training and experience, I am ill equipped to intelligently debate the limitations of science, *per se*. This has not been the intent of my examination during the preceding pages. I am a physician, who has, on occasion, utilized scientific principles, but I am not a scientist. My point is and has been that medicine utilizes many scientific principles, but is not, in fact, a scientific discipline. The conclusions that are often reached, as illustrated in the previous chapters, may be based on controversial or incomplete studies and from these conclusions recommendations are made by a consensus of expert panels and organizations that are not immune to influence peddling from industry, whose bottom line is not necessarily the public health.

Probably the principal motivation for this book is a desire to counter the chronic and persistent arrogance with which medical "experts"— be they radio or TV gurus; or professors at medical conferences; or the litany of alternative/complementary/functional medicine authors — smugly endorse universal recommendations regarding health care. They are as self-assured as those who quote "scripture" with the confidence of theologians. Most of what I will say in the following pages concerns what I perceive to be the overstatements of medical researchers and the clinicians who, while often not understanding the research itself, nonetheless accept the implications of that research.

The general public, including the educated, but not scientifically trained, regards science as eminently successful; and rightly so, as its successes have been impressive. Some of these notable successes over the past 100 years or so includes Banting and Best's discovery of insulin; Zworykin's invention of the television camera; and Flemings discovery of penicillin — all in the 1920s. Percy Julian's development of synthetic cortisone in 1948 and Watson, Crick and Franklin's discovery of the double helix structure of DNA in 1953 are just two examples of the extraordinary scientific accomplishments later in the twentieth century. Within the past 2 years we learned of some scientific discoveries that simply boggle the mind — including the creation of a mouse in Japan by using eggs derived from stem cells alone (1). In addition, a new developing study reports of a extraordinarily high tech female condom that not only blocks sperm but also emits an anti-HIV medication and then disappears (2).

Because of such impressive advances in medical research, pronouncements and recommendations made by the medical (research) community are often accepted as valid, without any skepticism, as they are presumed to be based upon science. There are several individuals who have devoted their lives to the study and critique of science's success including Thomas Kuhn and Paul Feyerabend, but they were referring primarily to the so-called "physical" sciences such as biology, chemistry, and physics. In *Against Method*, Feyerabend (3) states:

Science is only one of the many instruments people invented to cope with their surroundings. It is not the only one, it is not infallible, and it has become too powerful, too pushy, and too dangerous to be left on its own.

Note that he was speaking of the so-called "hard sciences", which have the capacity to intimidate many of us. Therefore imagine the considerable reservations that we justifiably might have regarding science's offspring, medicine. Unlike laboratory investigators in hard science, researchers attempting to study human beings have a difficult time taking under consideration all of the socio-economic, psychological, and genetic underpinnings that can influence how humans respond to experimental intervention. The argument is not that the randomized clinical trial is without value. On the contrary, it is probably the single most reliable tool for finding answers to clinical questions; however, to paraphrase Feyerabend, it is not the only tool, it is not infallible and it has, indeed become too prevalent as the sole determinant in making sweeping generalizations regarding the public's health. I would emphasize this because during the past 30 years I have listened to several professors of medicine pontificate that "the science has clearly shown…" when, in fact, the (medical) science rarely clearly shows anything, and can certainly never *conclusively* prove anything regarding the unstudied population.

It is not easy to say definitively what science *is*, but at the very least we can say that it is a human activity devised to answer questions, which involves observation, hypothesis generation, and testing through experimentation. Although, as science writer and educator, Sherry Seethaler says, "this view of science is oversimplified, incomplete, and sets people up for failure when they try to make sense of science in the real world " (4). Medicine, perhaps one of the noblest of human activities and, here, I am admittedly and unashamedly biased, is, when done well, an art which uses scientific principles. Its nobility is inherent in that its AIM is healing — physically and/or emotionally. The instruments used are not merely the technology that has become available during the last generation, but first and foremost, the gift of communication; the desire and ability to communicate with any patient irrespective of age, gender, or background. This idealized description may seem unfamiliar given the greater publicity given to the practitioner who is accused of insurance fraud, malpractice, or various forms of abuse. The techniques used by the physician committed to the above mentioned AIM are varied. They may use information derived from clinical trials, randomized or not; clinical experience; anecdotal information; or just "gut feeling," or intuition; which is so often vilified, but may nonetheless be appropriate when dealing with the *individual* before you. The consensus-driven dogma, which often passes for science may be helpful, but should be regarded as a possible guide, not as a required roadmap as to how to proceed.

In the introduction to his excellent book, *The Trouble With Physics*, Lee Smolin quotes Nobel Laureate, David Gross, who closed a conference devoted to hailing the progress made in one of the current controversial fields of theoretical physics, string theory, by saying "We don't know what we're talking about" (5). Now to be fair and accurate Gross had much more to say and because of the controversy regarding his statements he did offer clarification and expansion of his comments. My point is that it would be refreshing and unexpected to hear one of the thought leaders in medicine speak with such honesty about some of medicine's cherished views.

A certain degree of uncertainty is inevitable in all areas of life, for whatever is not personally experienced is essentially hearsay. However, in clinical medicine (caring for patients), uncertainty is the rule; it is what we do on a regular basis. When confronted with a patient's complaints, we have learned, beginning in medical school, to think in terms of a "differential diagnosis" which means considering the numerous possibilities which could explain the symptoms. There are an extraordinary number of diseases that are said to be "idiopathic," which means we don't know their cause. As physicians, we say "The cause is not known," implying that no one knows, which sounds less self defeating than "I don't know." Biopsies (taking a piece of tissue) are frequently "non-diagnostic", as are x-rays, and laboratory tests. All of the above are examples of how often we are faced with uncertainty when dealing with an individual patient sitting across from us, whom we presumably know much about. Imagine then the uncertainty we are faced with when we are expected to consider information acquired on individuals whom we have never met, know nothing about personally, who underwent testing under conditions which we can never confirm, and the results of the tests having been interpreted using statistical methods which we likely do not understand. It is easy to see how much of what we do is essentially faith-based. Add to all of this ambiguity, the phenomenon of biological variability — not everyone's chemistry, physiology, or body is the same. Different individuals have different responses to treatment, especially if the treatment is chemical. Over the years, I have had countless patients tell me that they were experiencing a side effect to a medication which the books would suggest they shouldn't be experiencing. Is it "all in their head?" as we often say? Possibly. Or is it that, given biological variability, their body is reacting unexpectedly?

When describing the aim or intention of evidence-based medicine it is usually defined in politically correct and comprehensive terms such as "a technique to combine a physician's clinical experience with the use of best available evidence and at the same time incorporating the patient's personal values." In other words, all the bases are covered; however, in practice, EBM usually means clinical decisions based on what is increasingly called "the science," which is deemed to be the randomized clinical trial(s). We have already discussed why this is a useful but flawed instrument.

Clearly the objectives of EBM are worthy — to provide the best evidence available in order to better treat the patient — to provide better outcomes. Whether this objective has been accomplished after at least a generation is subject to dispute ((6) (7)). There is an inherent ethical dilemma involved in trying to prove that EBM results in better outcomes. If the randomized trial is the gold standard — the best way to establish efficacy — how could we justify having a control group who is denied access to the evidence? Much of what we do is an attempt to minimize uncertainty. This attempt is often manifested in a tendency in medicine to be more proactive. The mantra in medicine is generally, "don't just stand there, do something," drug it, burn it (radiation), or cut it out." It would not be a stretch to state that physician specialty choices can reflect, at least indirectly, a desire to avoid or minimize uncertainty. Studies in the sociology and medical education literature have shown that surgeons have less of a tolerance of uncertainty or ambiguity than internists or psychiatrists ((8) (9)). There is little doubt, both anecdotally and in published surveys, that potential surgeons are attracted to the greater prospects or perceptions of being able to provide fixes with the scalpel rather than just "plodding through" with drug or talk therapy. In psychiatry, talk has given way to "psychopharmacology". It is not uncommon for patients to go to a psychiatrist (MD) for a prescription, but see a psychologist (Masters or Ph.D.) for talk therapy.

The gist of this chapter is what should be apparent to anyone who has lived at least to adulthood and that is the reality that virtually every aspect of life is filled with uncertainty. Those involved in the human activity of science appreciate this truism, even if the less informed and therefore naïve idolators of scientism, cannot. Those of us who have spent a lifetime involved in the magnificent but all too human activity of clinical medicine appreciate that virtually every day of our practice (and it's called practice for good reason) is filled with uncertainty. Our growing tendency to rely more on randomized clinical trials rather than expert opinion is an understandable attempt to provide greater certainty to what we think we know and the rationale behind how we manage our patient's concerns. However, the argument is that just because the randomized trial may be the single best instrument we have to assess efficacy on a broad scale, we must not fool ourselves into believing that its predictive power is greater than it is or can ever be. This is particularly important to appreciate in view of the myriad of factors that influence how individuals respond to different treatments. Given the extraordinary complexity of human beings and that the best of our study instruments are flawed, it therefore follows that a greater sense of humility is warranted.

References Cited

1. Vogel, G. and D. Normile, Reprogrammed Cells Earn Biologists Top Honor. *Science*, 2012. 338(6104): p. 178-179.
2. Hickey, H. Electrically spun fabric offers dual defense against pregnancy, HIV. UW Today 2012 [cited 2013 September 1]; Available from: http://www.washington.edu/news/2012/11/30/electrically-spun-fabric-offers-dual-defense-against-pregnancy-hiv/.
3. Feyerabend, P., *Against Method*. London: Verso, 2010. p. 164.
4. Seethaler, S., Lies, *Damned Lies, and Science: How to Sort Through the Noise Around Global Warming, the Latest Health Claims, and Other Scientific Controversies*. Upper Saddle River, N.J: FT Press, 2009. p. 3.
5. Smolin, L., *The Trouble with Physics: The Rise of String Theory, the Fall of a Science and What Comes Next*. London: Penguin, 2008. p. XV.
6. Krumholz, H.M., M.J. Radford, E.F. Ellerbeck, J. Hennen, T.P. Meehan, M. Petrillo, Y. Wang, and S.F. Jencks, Aspirin for secondary prevention after acute myocardial infarction in the elderly: prescribed use and outcomes. *Annals of Internal Medicine*, 1996. 124(3): p. 292-298.

7. Wong, J.H., J.M. Findlay, and M.E. Suarez-Almazor, Regional performance of carotid endarterectomy appropriateness, outcomes, and risk factors for complications. *Stroke*, 1997. 28(5): p. 891-898.

8. Ghosh, A., Understanding medical uncertainty: a primer for physicians. *JAPI*, 2004. 52: p. 739-742.

9. Gerrity, M.S., K.P. White, R.F. DeVellis, and R.S. Dittus, Physicians' reactions to uncertainty: refining the constructs and scales. *Motivation and Emotion*, 1995. 19(3): p. 175-191.

CHAPTER 11

The Need for Humility

MOST DEFINITIONS OF humility usually include wording such as "a state of being humble"(1), "a modest estimate of one's worth,"(2) or "the lack of pride."(3). Merriam-Webster also defines the opposite of humility as arrogance, a term that is often carries with it a negative connotation. However, we cannot assume that arrogance has a such a connotation in everyone's mind; In a 1980 essay by the late gastroenterologist and former editor of *The New England Journal of Medicine*, Franz Inglefinger, argued that arrogance, which he understood to involve elements of authoritarianism, paternalism, and domination, was "essential to good medical care" (4). In the interest of fairness, however, an explanation of what he meant, is necessary and I will attempt to clarify this later in the chapter.

In the major religious traditions, humility is an admirable and desirable trait. Humility is viewed in the Abrahamic monotheistic faiths — the big three — Judaism, Christianity, and Islam, as beneficial. According to Rabbi Dr. Louis Jacobs (1920-2006) a leader of conservative Judaism in the United Kingdom:

In the Jewish tradition, humility is among the greatest of the virtues, as its opposite, pride, is among the worst of the vices. Moses, the greatest of men, is described as the most humble: "Now the man Moses was very meek, above all the men that were on the face of the earth (Numbers 12:3)" The patriarch Abraham protests to God: "Behold now, I have taken upon me to speak unto the Lord, who am but dust and ashes (Genesis 18:27)"(5).

Jacobs further recounts the story of a man who comes to the leader of a Hasidic group and complains,

"All my life, he said, I have tried to follow the advice of the rabbis that one who runs away from fame will find that fame pursues him, and yet while I run away from fame, fame never seems to pursue me." The leader replied: "The trouble is that while you do run away from fame you are always looking over your shoulder to see if fame is chasing after you" (6).

In the Christian religion, it is said that humility is essential for being a true disciple of Christ. The New Testament is especially replete with numerous examples of the primacy of this virtue For example, Matt. 12:11; John 12:12–17; and Phil. 2:3. (7).

In the teachings of Islam, it is said that only one thing raises one man or woman above another and that is piety. True piety is said to be achievable only by cultivating a sense of humility (8). In the Quran (31:18) it is said that "God doesn't like an arrogant boaster"(9).

All of the above not withstanding, humility in the discipline of medicine often has been described as "a square peg in a round hole"(10). It is often perceived as being clearly out of place and a sign of weakness that can only damage the necessary confidence that a patient has in their doctor. The popular image of the doctor exemplified by most of the characters on the popular medical dramas on TV is that of a bold, confident, brilliant risk taker. They all seem to be saying, "I'm a surgeon, damn it, I save lives and I'm going to do this because it is the right thing to do." One almost wants to say, "yes, you are a surgeon and you often save lives, but where in the Hippocratic or any other oath does it say that you *have* to be an A-hole?"

June Tangney in the introduction to her paper on humility (11), states that it is a neglected virtue in the social and psychological sciences; imagine then the lack of respect with which the "virtue" is regarded by many of those who like to think that they are practicing scientific medicine. Contrary to the perception that humility is a sign of weakness and indecisiveness, Tangney suggests, "humility can denote a willingness to accurately assess oneself and one's limitations, the ability to acknowledge gaps in one's knowledge and demonstrate an openness to new ideas, contradictory information and advice" (12). This approach or attitude is appropriate because, as discussed in previous chapters, decisions made in medicine are almost always accompanied by uncertainty. Our knowledge base often is suspect. While the extraordinary accomplishments of medicine over the past 100 years — not just drug therapy and surgical procedures but also improvements in sanitation and nutrition — is justification for pride; however, we still need appreciate the opportunity we have been given to be so intimately involved in the lives of our patients.

Concerning Inglefinger's seeming endorsement of arrogance and his assertion that it is often essential to providing good medical care, he offered a personal anecdote as an illustration. When he was first diagnosed with cancer, he spoke with a number of colleagues regarding options for therapy. He and his family were given numerous opinions and approaches that ultimately created a great deal of anguish for him and his family. He was also disadvantaged by the fact that he was, as a gastroenterologist, an "expert" in the very type of cancer which he had. He says that he received from physician friends throughout the country "a barrage of well-intentioned but contradictory advice." Can you imagine what the nonphysician, non-expert patient must feel when confronted with having to make these decisions?

"Finally, when the pangs of indecision had become nearly intolerable, one wise physician friend said, 'what you need is a doctor.' He was telling me to forget the information I already had and the information

I was receiving from many quarters, and to seek instead a person who would dominate, who would tell me what to do, who would in a paternalistic manner assume responsibility for my care (13)."

This is not quite what many of us have in mind when we speak of arrogance in medicine. Given the circumstances of the above dilemma, I would be more inclined to refer to this as welcomed benign paternalism. The disease which I am referring to — that of lack of humility and an exaggerated sense of self importance — results in a failure to appreciate the very tenuousness of the conclusions we draw from the medical literature and consequently, the recommendations we make to our patients, as well as the general public. It is my hope that this text can make at least a modest contribution to a greater appreciation of the inherent and unavoidable uncertainty in what we are told, what we think we understand and encourage us to avoid taking dogmatic positions regarding the treatment and management of human beings.

In addition to exposing the folly of medical dogma, changes in medical education are critical to minimizing the acceptance of the myths of medical certainty. To acquire this sense of humility, to be better able to assess our limitations, as Tangney suggests, and acknowledge the gaps in our knowledge, some changes will be necessary in the way we train health care providers, especially physicians. The Association of American Medical Colleges (AAMC), the 137-year-old organization that represents all 141 accredited US and 17 accredited Canadian medical schools has recognized the need to grow and develop in response to an increasingly diverse patient population. This is directly in keeping with its mission of advancing medical education. Some states, namely New Jersey and California are already requiring physicians to take continuing courses in what is called cultural competence. These classes are designed to better assist them to relate to a diverse patient population; the AAMC has recommended that a "cultural competence educational program ultimately be effectively integrated throughout all years of medical school" (14). There will no doubt be resistance to these mandates. I argue, however, that a culturally competent physician is more likely to be open to diversity of opinion and people, more reflective and less arrogant. This of course remains to be demonstrated. There also needs to be some training in research methodology and particularly its limitations. One should not have to wait until graduate school, after medical school (as I did) to learn something about the language of research; *i.e.* biostatistics and epidemiology. In so far as pharmacology (the study of drugs) is a basic part of the curriculum of all medical schools, nutrition and environmental science should also be part of every curriculum so that the developing physician can begin to appreciate other possibilities of disease causation and treatment.

It is often presumed that only certain "types" of individuals are attracted to the medical profession and sought after by the admission committees of medical schools (15). The bias generally seems to be to accept students with a strong background in the "hard sciences" and the highest of scores on the Medical College Aptitude Test (MCAT) (16), however, it may be more important to recruit students who have demonstrated competence with handling some basic science but who also show competence in and an affinity for the humanities and social sciences, beyond basic requirements. The very good news is that there is a growing appreciation that the non-traditional student can be considered without compromising relevant academic standards, and more importantly, good patient care.

In 1987, The Humanities and Medicine Program (HuMed) was established at Mount Sinai School of Medicine in New York City (17). They offered guaranteed admission to qualified second and third year college students who were majoring in the social sciences and humanities, provided they went on to complete their bachelor's degree. Once accepted into the program, the students had to maintain a B+ average. They were not required to take the MCAT or organic chemistry, physics and calculus, a few of the more rigorous traditional premed courses. After completing the third year of college they were required to spend an 8-week summer term at Mount Sinai where they were exposed to the various medical specialties and attend seminars in bioethics, health policy, and emotional and clinical treatment for patients living with serious illness, so-called palliative care. The students also took an abbreviated course in the principles of organic chemistry and physics as they relate to medicine. Once completing their undergraduate degree they were encouraged to take a year off before starting medical school. The HuMed program was initially a pilot project with a small percentage of students (approx. 12–15%) accepted each year. In 2010, a study was completed and published comparing the medical school performance outcomes of the HuMed students with their classmates who were more traditionally prepared. The goal was to determine if pre-med requirements could predict success in medical school. The conclusion was that the HuMed students performed at the same level as their classmates. The program was deemed so successful that beginning in 2013–2014, Mount Sinai started recruiting half of each class from this non-traditional pool in their second year of college and offering them guaranteed acceptance if they fulfill the aforementioned criteria.

Admittedly, this may appear to be a shameful plug for my "type" as I was a political science major who worked as a social worker before attending medical school. One of the major challenges for me as a freshman medical student with a nontraditional background was understanding what my first semester studies had to do with what I ultimately wanted to do —take care of people. I will never forget the words of our well-meaning anatomy professor, who stated during the first week of class, "you will not likely retain more than 25% of what you will learn this semester." This suggested to me and was later confirmed, that much of what we were involved in was essentially mindless memorization of facts for the purpose of passing tests and moving on to the next level. Much of the first two years of my medical school was an obstacle course at least partially designed to weed out students.

I distinctly remember a few of my classmates who had traditional basic science backgrounds, appeared to be intelligent and compassionate young men and women, but who, for whatever reasons — not good test takers, perhaps — could not pass gross anatomy or biochemistry and were subsequently asked to leave. Approximately twenty years later, my daughter attended another medical school where it was not uncommon at that time for approximately twenty percent of the freshman class to either repeat the first year or be asked to leave. Given the backgrounds of most of these students at the time, this suggests that something was and is seriously wrong with either the recruitment or educational process. This is why the HUMed, now called FlexMed program offers a refreshing and sensible alternative to medical education, which will hopefully become, in time, the traditional approach to medical education.

In an article in *The New England Journal of Medicine*, Dr. David Muller, chair of the department of medical education at Mount Sinai stated that "information technology has made memorizing vast amounts of content unnecessary" (18). He further pointed out that "the current (traditional) model has perpetuated premed syndrome; a culture of aggressive competition for grades that conflicts with the precepts of medical professionalism, academic and intellectual rigor, creative thinking, collaboration, and social conscience" (19).

Most of this text was designed to give the student or just thoughtful reader a perspective, a basis upon which to look at medical recommendations that are made. The message for current and future health care providers, however, is the hope that, irrespective of academic background, we can still appreciate the absence of certainty in the real world and the consequent need for humility in our dealings with human beings, particularly those who honor us by coming to us for care.

References Cited

1. Merriam-Webster Inc., *The Merriam-Webster Dictionary.* 2005, Springfield, Mass.: Merriam-Webster.
2. Flexner, S.B., J.M. Stein, and P.Y. Su, *The Random House Dictionary.* Classic ed. 1983, New York: Random House.
3. Morris, W., *The American Heritage Dictionary of the English language.* 1971, New York: American Heritage Pub. Co..
4. Ingelfinger, F.J., Arrogance. *The New England Journal of Medicine,* 1980. **303**(26): p. 1507.
5. Jacobs, L., *The Jewish Religion: A Companion.* 1995, Oxford: Oxford University Press
6. Ibid.
7. Zondervan Publishing House (Grand Rapids Mich.), *The Holy Bible.* 2007, Grand Rapids, Mich.: Zondervan.
8. Stacey, A. *Humility.* IslamReligion.com 2008 [cited 2013 October 19]; Available from: http://www.islamreligion.com/articles/1693/.
9. Ali, A.Y., *The Holy Quran : Text, Translation & Commentary.* New ed. 1983, Lahore: Sh. M. Ashraf.
10. Coulehan, J., On humility. *Annals of Internal Medicine,* 2010. **153**(3): p. 200-201.
11. Tangney, J.P., Humility: Theoretical perspectives, empirical findings and directions for future research. *Journal of Social and Clinical Psychology,* 2000. **19**(1): p. 70-82.
12. Ibid.
13. Ingelfinger, F.J.
14. AAMC, Cultural Competence Education, 2005.
15. Chen, P., The changing face of medical school admissions, in The New York Times May 2, 2013: New York.
16. Hartocollis, A., Getting Into medical school without hard sciences, in New York Times June 29, 2010: New York.
17. Muller, D. and N. Kase, Challenging traditional premedical

requirements as predictors of success in medical school: The Mount Sinai School of Medicine Humanities and Medicine Program. *Academic Medicine*, 2010. **85**(8): p. 1378-1383.

18. Muller, D., Reforming Premedical Education—Out with the Old, In with the New. *New England Journal of Medicine*, 2013. **368**(17): p. 1567-1569.

19. Muller, D., Reforming Premedical Education—Out with the Old, In with the New. *New England Journal of Medicine*, 2013. **368**(17): p. 1567-1569.

"One Never Knows, do one?" - Fat's Waller

Index

I

Inglefinger, Franz 124

Institute of Medicine 17

J

Jacobs, Louis (Rabbi) 124, 125

Japanese Migration Studies 85

Jenner, Edward 67, 68

K

Kendrick, Malcolm 89, 91

Keys, Ancel 84, 90

Kuhn, Thomas 11, 117

L

Lind, James 12

Louis, Pierre 14

LSD 72

M

Mahareshi, Mahesh Yogi 102

Maxwell, James Clerk 22

Medical Research Council (MRC) 15

Morgantaler, Abraham 39

N

National Cancer Institute 58, 59

Null, Gary 103, 104, 107

Null Hypothesis 27, 28

O

Office of Technology Assessment (OTA) 16

Oz, Mehmet (Dr.) 104

W

Z

CPSIA information can be obtained
at www.ICGtesting.com
Printed in the USA
BVOW10s0532220717

489698BV00007B/151/P